The Complete Obesity Fix Cookbook Inspired by Dr James DiNicolantonio's Teachings

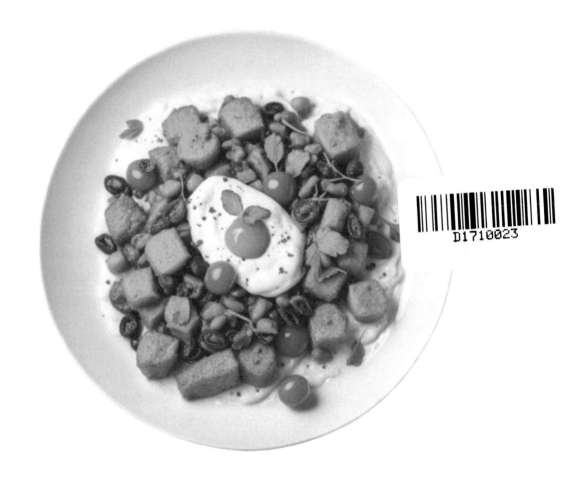

Quick and Easy Healthy Recipes for Lasting Weight Loss and Vibrant Energy

Michelle C. Huff

Disclaimer

This book is intended for informational and educational purposes only. The content is not meant to be a substitute for professional medical advice, diagnosis, or treatment. Always seek the guidance of your physician or other qualified health provider with any questions you may have regarding a medical condition or dietary plan. The author, Michelle C. Huff, is not responsible for any adverse effects, consequences, or damages resulting from the use or application of the information in this book.

The recipes and nutritional information provided are based on general recommendations and should be adapted to suit individual needs. Results may vary, and it is important to consult with a healthcare professional before making any significant changes to your diet or lifestyle, particularly if you have any pre-existing medical conditions.

Introduction

The world is facing a surge in obesity, affecting all age groups, social backgrounds, and regions. What was once a rare issue confined to specific populations has become a global health crisis, impacting billions of people. But obesity is not simply a matter of excess body weight; it's a condition that penetrates every aspect of health. It sets off a cascade of issues, significantly raising the risk of chronic diseases like diabetes, heart disease, and certain types of cancer. These illnesses aren't isolated; they're intertwined with our quality of life and longevity. As obesity rates rise, so do healthcare costs, burdening not only individuals but also national healthcare systems worldwide.

In recent decades, obesity has transitioned from an uncommon problem to one of the most prevalent health issues of our time. It's easy to think of obesity as a simple matter of eating too much and moving too little, but this oversimplification fails to capture the full picture. Obesity doesn't emerge overnight. Instead, it's the cumulative result of years of subtle shifts in lifestyle, diet, and even societal norms. Understanding how these changes took place provides insight into why so many people struggle with weight and why traditional weight loss advice often fails.

The Underlying Causes of Obesity

Modern life has brought unparalleled convenience, especially in the way we eat. Our lives have sped up, and food companies have adapted by providing quick, processed, and calorie-dense options that are easy to overeat and often nutritionally poor. These foods are engineered to be hyper-palatable—meaning they're designed to be irresistible, with the perfect balance of sugar, fat, and salt that makes it difficult to stop eating. They bypass the body's natural satiety signals, leading us to eat more than we need.

On top of that, these foods are inexpensive and widely available, making them an easy choice in a world where time is limited, and fresh foods can be more costly and less convenient. This shift in diet has created a disconnect between the food we eat and the nutrients our bodies need. Rather than nourishing us, these foods often leave us feeling unsatisfied, leading to more frequent cravings and, ultimately, weight gain.

Another significant contributor to obesity is the drastic reduction in physical activity. As technology has advanced, physical labor has decreased, with many people spending hours in front of screens, either for work or leisure. Our ancestors were constantly on the move, hunting, gathering, and working physically to survive. Today, however, many people lead sedentary lives, relying on modern conveniences like cars and elevators that reduce the need for movement. This lack of physical activity creates an energy imbalance where the body stores more calories as fat rather than burning them for energy.

Biological and Psychological Factors

Biology also plays a critical role. Hormones like insulin, leptin, and ghrelin regulate hunger and satiety, but a high-sugar, processed diet can disrupt these systems. For instance, high sugar intake can lead to insulin resistance, which over time can promote fat storage, especially around the abdomen. Similarly, leptin, the hormone responsible for signaling fullness, can become ineffective when exposed to frequent spikes in insulin and high-calorie foods. This condition, known as leptin resistance, makes it difficult for the body to recognize when it has had enough, leading to overeating.

Psychological factors are equally significant. Stress, for example, triggers the release of cortisol, a hormone that can promote fat storage and increase cravings for high-calorie foods. Additionally, many people use food as a coping mechanism, leading to "emotional eating" where food is used for comfort rather than nourishment. This can create a vicious cycle, where overeating leads to weight gain, which can then lead to negative emotions like shame or guilt—emotions that people often try to soothe with more food.

Social and Environmental Influences

Our environment and social setting also have a profound impact. In many societies, food is used as a social tool, present in celebrations, gatherings, and even work meetings. This constant exposure to food, combined with social pressure, can make it hard to resist overeating, even when we aren't hungry. In addition, urban areas often have "food deserts," where access to fresh fruits and vegetables is limited, but fast food and convenience stores are plentiful. This lack of access to healthy food options further exacerbates the problem.

The Necessity of a Comprehensive Approach

Obesity is a complex condition influenced by a range of factors, from the physical and biological to the social and psychological. This complexity is why traditional weight-loss approaches that focus solely on cutting calories or increasing exercise often don't work in the long term. Instead, a more comprehensive approach that addresses all these underlying factors is needed. Understanding these roots allows individuals to make more informed choices about their health and equips them with practical strategies that address not just symptoms, but the core of the issue.

In the chapters that follow, we'll explore each of these factors in detail and discuss effective, science-based approaches for regaining control over weight and health. This knowledge is the first step toward breaking free from the cycle of obesity and setting the foundation for sustainable well-being.

Chapter 1
Understanding Obesity

Obesity is a multifaceted condition that cannot be reduced to simply "eating too much" or "not exercising enough." It's a complex interplay of dietary habits, hormonal signals, lifestyle choices, and even environmental factors that work together to influence how our bodies store and use energy. In a world where highly palatable, calorie-dense foods are abundant and movement is increasingly minimized, maintaining a healthy weight requires a deep understanding of the mechanisms driving weight gain.

Beyond Willpower: The Biological Basis of Obesity

When discussing obesity, it's essential to recognize that biology plays a foundational role. Our bodies evolved to survive in environments where food was scarce, not abundant. In those conditions, storing energy as fat was advantageous, providing reserves that could be drawn upon during times of scarcity. However, in modern times, this evolutionary trait has turned against us. The body's natural inclination to store energy in the form of fat persists, even when food is readily available. Additionally, certain individuals may have a genetic predisposition that makes them more efficient at storing fat, putting them at an even higher risk of obesity.

Several hormones regulate hunger, satiety, and fat storage, creating a delicate balance that our modern diet can easily disrupt. Insulin, for instance, is a hormone that helps regulate blood sugar levels and signals the body to store excess energy as fat. When we consume a diet high in refined sugars and carbohydrates, insulin levels spike more frequently. Over time, this can lead to insulin resistance, a condition where the body's cells become less responsive to insulin's effects. This resistance forces the body to produce even more insulin to manage blood sugar, creating a vicious cycle that encourages the body to store more fat, especially in the abdominal region.

Another critical hormone, leptin, signals the brain when the body has stored enough fat, prompting us to stop eating. However, as with insulin, a high-calorie, processed diet can lead to leptin resistance, where the brain no longer responds appropriately to leptin signals. This condition makes it difficult for people to feel full, leading to overeating. Thus, the body's hormonal system, designed to regulate appetite and maintain energy balance, becomes disrupted, making weight control increasingly challenging.

The Role of Processed Foods and Overeating

In today's food landscape, processed foods dominate. These foods are often high in refined sugars, unhealthy fats, and additives, all of which are designed to make them taste good and trigger the reward centers in our brains. They're engineered to be hyper-palatable, which means they are nearly impossible to resist and often lead to overeating. Unlike whole foods, which are rich in fiber and nutrients, processed foods are absorbed rapidly, causing quick spikes and drops in blood sugar levels. This cycle leaves us feeling hungry soon after eating, even though we've consumed plenty of calories.

Moreover, these foods bypass the body's natural satiety mechanisms, meaning they don't trigger the same fullness signals that whole foods would. This is particularly true for foods high in sugar and fat, like pastries, chips, and sugary drinks. These items can be consumed in large quantities without the body's usual cues to stop eating. The more frequently we consume these foods, the more we train our bodies to seek out high-calorie, nutrient-poor options, contributing to a pattern of overeating.

Lifestyle Factors: Sedentary Living and Energy Imbalance

Our increasingly sedentary lifestyle compounds the challenges of maintaining a healthy weight. Many people today spend the majority of their day sitting—at work, in cars, and at home. Physical activity, which helps burn calories and regulates metabolic health, has decreased significantly, contributing to a state of chronic energy imbalance. When we consume more calories than we burn, the excess energy is stored as fat.

Physical activity does more than just burn calories; it also supports the body's ability to use insulin effectively and maintain a healthy metabolism. Regular movement increases muscle mass, which in turn raises the body's basal metabolic rate, or the number of calories burned at rest. A higher muscle mass makes it easier to maintain a healthy weight, as the body naturally expends more energy throughout the day. However, when physical activity is minimal, muscle mass declines, the metabolism slows, and the body becomes more prone to storing fat. This is why physical inactivity is one of the primary lifestyle factors contributing to obesity.

The Cycle of Weight Gain: A Challenging Pattern to Break

When the body's energy balance, hormones, and eating habits are disrupted, a challenging cycle of weight gain emerges. Processed foods promote overeating, hormonal imbalances make it harder to feel full, and physical inactivity slows down metabolism. Each of these factors reinforces the others, making it difficult for individuals to break free from the cycle of weight gain.

For example, someone who eats a diet high in refined sugars might experience frequent insulin spikes, leading to insulin resistance and increased fat storage. This additional weight may make physical activity more challenging, further reducing calorie expenditure and leading to more weight gain. At the same time, the constant consumption of high-calorie foods blunts the effectiveness of hormones like leptin, making it even harder to resist cravings and establish healthy eating patterns.

Moving Toward Solutions

Despite these challenges, understanding the various factors driving obesity provides a roadmap for effective intervention. By recognizing that weight gain is not simply a matter of willpower, we can approach weight management in a more compassionate and scientifically grounded way. Rather than focusing solely on calorie restriction or exercise, a successful approach to weight loss considers the entire system: improving dietary choices, rebalancing hormones, and gradually increasing physical activity.

In the following sections, we'll explore practical strategies to tackle each of these issues individually and create an environment that supports long-term health. Breaking the cycle of obesity is possible with a comprehensive plan that targets the root causes of weight gain and helps the body find a healthy balance once again.

Chapter 2
The Role of Food

Food is more than fuel; it's a powerful force that shapes our metabolism, influences our hormones, and dictates how we store or burn fat. Different types of foods have vastly different effects on the body, particularly when it comes to weight management. Some foods drive fat storage and disrupt metabolic health, while others can support energy balance and nourish our cells.

In the modern diet, certain categories of food—namely sugars, refined carbohydrates, and certain fats—are leading culprits in the obesity epidemic. These foods not only provide excess calories but also cause biochemical shifts that make weight management even more difficult. Understanding how these foods affect the body can empower us to make choices that better align with our health and weight goals.

Sugars: Fueling Cravings and Fat Storage

Sugar, particularly refined sugar, is one of the most problematic ingredients in the modern diet. Not only does it provide "empty calories" (calories without nutrients), but it also has a unique ability to disrupt our body's natural hunger and energy systems.

When we consume sugar, it rapidly raises blood glucose levels. This spike triggers the pancreas to release insulin, a hormone that helps cells absorb glucose for energy. However, when we consume sugar frequently or in large amounts, insulin levels remain high for prolonged periods. This constant exposure to high insulin can lead to insulin resistance, a condition where cells no longer respond effectively to insulin, forcing the body to produce even more insulin. Insulin resistance encourages the body to store more energy as fat, particularly in the abdominal area, which is associated with a higher risk of chronic diseases like diabetes and cardiovascular issues.

Moreover, sugar affects the brain's reward system, creating a feedback loop that can lead to cravings and overeating. When we eat sugar, it releases dopamine, a neurotransmitter associated with pleasure and reward. The more frequently we consume sugar, the more we reinforce this dopamine pathway, conditioning the brain to crave sugar regularly. Over time, this can lead to a cycle of cravings that's difficult to break, fueling both overeating and weight gain.

Refined Carbohydrates: Rapid Energy with Lasting Impact

Refined carbohydrates, like those found in white bread, pasta, pastries, and other processed foods, are another significant driver of weight gain. Unlike whole grains, which contain fiber and nutrients, refined carbs are stripped of their beneficial components, leaving behind a product that quickly breaks down into glucose.

When we consume refined carbs, they're rapidly digested and absorbed, causing a quick spike in blood sugar. This surge leads to a corresponding spike in insulin, similar to the effect seen with sugar. However, the rapid breakdown of these foods means that blood sugar levels quickly drop again after the initial spike, leading to energy crashes that often prompt further cravings. This "roller coaster" effect on blood sugar not only promotes fat storage but also leads to more frequent hunger and overeating.

Refined carbs are also low in fiber, a critical nutrient that slows digestion and helps us feel full. Without fiber, these foods fail to trigger the satiety signals that whole foods do, making it easier to consume larger portions without feeling satisfied. The combination of low satiety, rapid digestion, and frequent insulin spikes makes refined carbs a potent factor in the development of obesity, especially when consumed regularly.

Fats: The Good, the Bad, and the Misunderstood

For many years, dietary fat was blamed for weight gain, but not all fats are equal. While some types of fat can contribute to inflammation and fat storage, others play essential roles in metabolism, hormone regulation, and even fat burning.

Unhealthy Fats: Trans fats and certain omega-6 fats found in processed foods and vegetable oils are the types most closely linked with weight gain and inflammation. Trans fats, in particular, are artificially created fats found in many processed foods, such as baked goods and margarine. These fats are not only harmful to heart health but can also interfere with metabolic processes, promoting fat storage and increasing the risk of obesity. Similarly, omega-6 fats, while essential in small amounts, can contribute to inflammation when consumed in excess, particularly when they're out of balance with anti-inflammatory omega-3 fats.

Healthy Fats: In contrast, monounsaturated fats (found in olive oil, avocados, and nuts) and polyunsaturated fats (such as omega-3s found in fatty fish) are beneficial for health and weight management. These fats help reduce inflammation, support metabolic health, and can even promote satiety, making it easier to control calorie intake. Fats like these are digested more slowly than carbohydrates, helping to stabilize blood sugar and reduce hunger between meals. Including healthy fats in the diet can support a balanced metabolism and reduce the likelihood of overeating, especially when paired with fiber-rich foods.

Choosing Foods that Support Metabolic Health

While certain foods disrupt metabolism and promote weight gain, others support energy balance and help manage weight effectively. Whole, unprocessed foods, including vegetables, lean proteins, healthy fats, and whole grains, provide the nutrients and fiber needed for a stable metabolism.

Fiber, in particular, is a powerful ally in weight management. Foods high in fiber, like vegetables, fruits, legumes, and whole grains, slow digestion, helping to keep blood sugar levels stable and prolonging feelings of fullness. Fiber also feeds beneficial gut bacteria, which play a role in metabolism, inflammation, and overall health. By prioritizing fiber-rich foods, we can support both weight management and overall well-being.

In addition to fiber, protein is another important component. Protein helps regulate hunger hormones, keeping us full longer and reducing the temptation to snack. Lean sources of protein, such as fish, chicken, beans, and tofu, support muscle health and metabolic rate, especially when combined with regular physical activity.

By focusing on these types of foods, we can create a diet that supports the body's natural ability to regulate weight. Unlike diets that rely on strict calorie counting or food restriction, a balanced diet rich in whole foods promotes a healthy metabolism, stable energy levels, and a reduced likelihood of cravings.

Balancing Hormones through Food Choices

Food choices directly impact the body's hormonal landscape, and by making strategic adjustments, we can support hormone balance and improve weight control. A diet that's lower in sugar and refined carbohydrates, for instance, reduces the frequency of insulin spikes, helping the body become more sensitive to insulin over time. This not only promotes weight loss but also reduces the risk of developing type 2 diabetes.

Additionally, consuming anti-inflammatory foods like leafy greens, fatty fish, nuts, and seeds can help balance other hormones, like cortisol, which is often elevated in response to stress. Elevated cortisol levels can lead to increased fat storage, particularly around the abdomen. By choosing foods that support hormonal health, we create a more stable internal environment that is conducive to maintaining a healthy weight.

Understanding the role of different foods in metabolism and weight gain is essential for making informed dietary choices. By minimizing intake of sugars, refined carbs, and unhealthy fats, while focusing on fiber, protein, and healthy fats, we can better support our body's natural mechanisms for weight management. This approach isn't about restriction or deprivation; it's about making choices that nourish the body and promote lasting health.

In the following sections, we'll explore how to structure a diet that is not only satisfying but also sustainable, setting the stage for successful long-term weight management.

Chapter 3
Creating a Balanced Diet

A balanced diet isn't about rigid restriction or deprivation; it's about choosing foods that nourish and sustain, keeping the body fueled, satiated, and energized. The foundation of a balanced diet lies in whole, nutrient-dense foods that provide the fiber, protein, and healthy fats needed to stabilize blood sugar, manage appetite, and reduce cravings. By focusing on these principles, we create an approach that's not only effective for weight management but also promotes long-term health and well-being.

The key to creating a balanced diet is to prioritize satisfaction and sustainability. Food should be enjoyable, and a healthy diet shouldn't feel like a constant battle against hunger or cravings. When we eat foods that nourish without spiking blood sugar, we support the body's natural hunger and fullness signals, making it easier to eat in a way that feels satisfying and sustainable over the long term.

The Core Elements of a Balanced Diet

- **Fiber-Rich Foods:** Fiber is one of the most powerful tools for managing hunger and supporting metabolic health. It slows down digestion, which helps stabilize blood sugar and prolongs feelings of fullness. High-fiber foods like vegetables, fruits, legumes, and whole grains provide bulk to meals without adding a lot of calories, making it easier to eat mindfully and avoid overeating. Additionally, fiber feeds beneficial gut bacteria, which play a role in weight management, immune function, and inflammation control.
- **Protein:** Protein is another cornerstone of a balanced diet, as it has a powerful impact on satiety and metabolism. When we consume protein, it triggers the release of appetite-regulating hormones, helping us feel full for longer and reducing the likelihood of snacking between meals. Protein also helps preserve lean muscle mass, which is important for maintaining a healthy metabolism. Lean protein sources such as fish, chicken, beans, and tofu are excellent choices, providing essential amino acids without excess calories or unhealthy fats.

- **Healthy Fats:** Fats have been unfairly demonized in the past, but certain fats are essential for health and can actually support weight management. Healthy fats, like those found in olive oil, nuts, seeds, and avocados, provide lasting energy and contribute to satiety, making it easier to avoid overeating. These fats are also anti-inflammatory and support hormonal balance, which is crucial for overall health. Including a moderate amount of healthy fats in each meal can help create balanced, satisfying meals that prevent cravings.
- **Minimizing Processed Foods:** Processed foods, particularly those high in sugar and refined carbs, are engineered to be hyper-palatable and often lead to overeating. These foods can disrupt blood sugar levels, leading to energy crashes and cravings shortly after eating. By limiting processed foods and focusing instead on whole foods, we avoid these spikes and crashes, creating a more stable energy profile throughout the day. Whole foods like vegetables, lean proteins, and whole grains help the body maintain a steady release of energy, supporting mood and reducing the temptation to reach for sugary or high-calorie snacks.

Structuring Balanced Meals

When building balanced meals, it's helpful to think in terms of food groups and proportions. Each meal should ideally include a mix of fiber, protein, and healthy fats, with a focus on keeping it colorful, varied, and enjoyable.

- **Start with Vegetables or Fiber-Rich Foods:** Vegetables and other fiber-rich foods should make up a significant portion of each meal. They are low in calories but high in volume, allowing you to eat a satisfying amount without excessive calories. Leafy greens, broccoli, carrots, bell peppers, and legumes are excellent choices that provide fiber, vitamins, and minerals.
- **Add a Lean Protein Source:** Next, include a serving of lean protein, such as chicken, fish, eggs, tofu, or legumes. Protein helps stabilize blood sugar levels and keeps you feeling full longer. It's also beneficial to incorporate plant-based proteins like lentils and chickpeas, which provide fiber along with protein for an extra satiating effect.
- **Include Healthy Fats:** Adding a source of healthy fat to your meal can increase satiety and improve nutrient absorption. Options like avocado, nuts, seeds, and olive oil provide essential fatty acids that help balance hormones and reduce inflammation. Just remember that fats are calorie-dense, so a little goes a long way; a few slices of avocado, a sprinkle of nuts, or a drizzle of olive oil can be sufficient.
- **Opt for Whole Grains or Starchy Vegetables:** If you're including grains or starches in

- your meal, choose whole grains or nutrient-dense starchy vegetables. Foods like quinoa, brown rice, sweet potatoes, and squash provide a steady source of energy without causing sharp spikes in blood sugar. These complex carbs are higher in fiber than their refined counterparts, promoting satiety and helping regulate blood sugar levels.
- **Stay Hydrated:** While it's easy to overlook, hydration plays a crucial role in appetite regulation and metabolic health. Drinking water or herbal teas throughout the day supports digestion and helps prevent false hunger signals that may actually be thirst. Starting meals with a glass of water can also help with portion control and satiety.

Reducing Cravings with Balanced Nutrition

One of the primary challenges in weight management is managing cravings, which are often driven by fluctuations in blood sugar and hormone levels. A balanced diet helps stabilize these levels, reducing the intensity and frequency of cravings. By choosing whole foods and including a combination of fiber, protein, and healthy fats, we can keep blood sugar steady and prevent the rapid rises and falls that lead to cravings.

Additionally, prioritizing nutrient-dense foods helps ensure the body receives the vitamins, minerals, and antioxidants it needs to function optimally. When the body is properly nourished, it's less likely to send out "hunger" signals in the form of cravings, especially for nutrient-poor foods like sweets and highly processed snacks.

Finding Enjoyment in Healthy Choices

Eating a balanced diet shouldn't mean sacrificing enjoyment. Restriction often leads to feelings of deprivation, which can make it harder to stick to healthy habits over the long term. Instead, a balanced approach encourages flexibility and satisfaction.

This can mean finding healthier versions of foods you love or incorporating small indulgences in a way that feels balanced. For example, instead of completely eliminating desserts, you might choose a small serving of dark chocolate or a homemade treat made with natural sweeteners. These choices allow you to enjoy food without derailing your health goals.

Experimenting with flavors, textures, and recipes can also make balanced eating more enjoyable. Herbs, spices, and various cooking techniques can add depth to meals, making them feel more satisfying and diverse. Cooking at home is another great way to create meals that align with your health goals while allowing for creativity and control over ingredients.

Long-Term Benefits of a Balanced Diet

A balanced diet offers numerous long-term benefits beyond weight management. By consistently choosing nutrient-dense foods, we support all aspects of health—from immune function to cognitive well-being and energy levels. A diet rich in whole foods has been shown to reduce inflammation, lower the risk of chronic diseases, and support a healthy gut microbiome, which is increasingly recognized as a key player in weight management and overall health.

Building balanced meals that are enjoyable and sustainable creates a positive relationship with food, reducing the likelihood of restrictive dieting and "yo-yo" weight cycling. When healthy eating feels achievable and satisfying, it becomes easier to make it a permanent lifestyle rather than a temporary fix.

The Obesity Fix Recipes

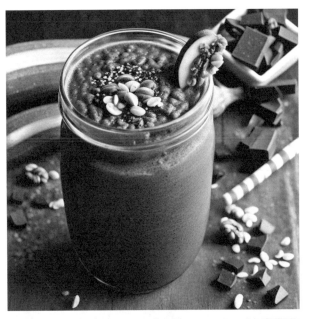

CHOCOLATE-ZUCCHINI SMOOTHIE

PREP TIME: 5 minutes SERVES 1

Ingredients

- ½ cup nonfat milk (or nondairy alternative)
- ½ zucchini, coarsely chopped
- ½ frozen banana
- 1 tablespoon cacao powder
- 1 teaspoon cacao nibs
- 2 tablespoons walnuts
- 1 teaspoon maple syrup
- 1 tablespoon rolled oats
- 1 tablespoon ground flaxseed
- ¼ cup plain nonfat Greek yogurt

Directions

- Fill the blender with the milk. Add the banana, rolled oats, flaxseed, yogurt, walnuts, cacao powder, cacao nibs, and maple syrup.
- Blend until the consistency you want is achieved, 30 to 60 seconds. If desired, thin with extra milk.

PER SERVING: Calories: 334; Total fat: 15g; Saturated fat: 2g; Sodium: 97mg; Carbohydrates: 41g; Fiber: 8g; Protein: 17g; Calcium: 281mg; Potassium: 1,052mg

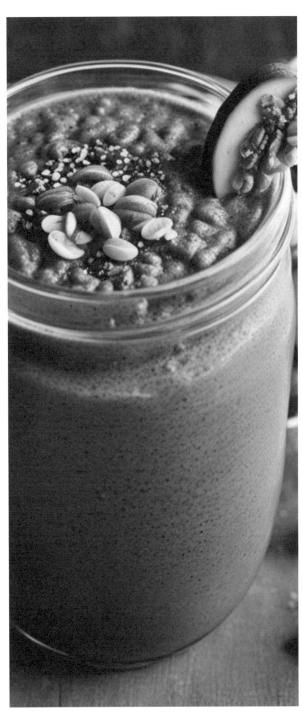

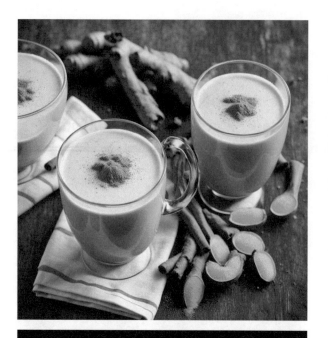

GOLDEN MILK SMOOTHIE

PREP TIME: 5 minutes SERVES 1

Ingredients

- ¼ cup nonfat milk
- 1 cup frozen mango
- ½ frozen banana
- ¾ cup plain kefir
- 1 teaspoon honey
- 1 teaspoon ground turmeric
- ½ teaspoon ground cinnamon
- 1 teaspoon ground flaxseed
- ¼ teaspoon ground ginger
- Pinch cayenne or freshly ground black pepper (optional)

Directions

- Fill the blender with the milk. Add the ginger, flaxseed, turmeric, cinnamon, kefir, honey, banana, mango, and cayenne, if using.
- Blend until the consistency you want is achieved, 30 to 60 seconds.

PER SERVING: Calories: 296; Total fat: 6g; Saturated fat: 3g; Sodium: 86mg; Carbohydrates: 56g; Fiber: 6g; Protein: 9g; Calcium: 270mg; Potassium: 873mg

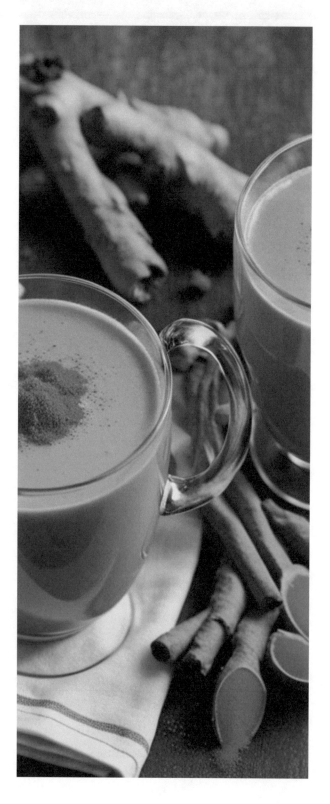

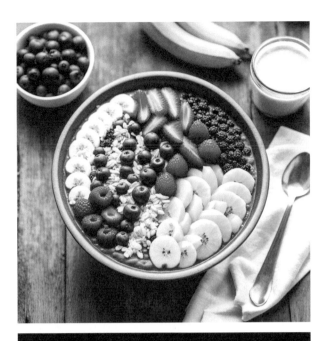

AÇAI SMOOTHIE BOWL

PREP TIME: 10 minutes SERVES 1 or 2

Ingredients

- 1 frozen açai packet
- ½ cup frozen mixed berries
- ½ frozen banana
- ½ cup frozen cauliflower florets
- ¾ cup plain nonfat Greek yogurt
- 1 tablespoon hemp seeds
- 1 tablespoon chia seeds
- 2 tablespoons rolled oats
- 1 tablespoon nut or seed butter
- ¼ cup unsweetened almond milk
- Granola, nuts, seeds, and/or fruit, for topping (optional)

Directions

- To soften the frozen açai package, run it under hot water for five seconds. Avoid defrosting.
- The açai, berries, banana, cauliflower, yogurt, chia seeds, hemp seeds, rolled oats, nut butter, and almond milk should all be combined in a high-speed blender.
- Using a rubber spatula or tamper to push down the ingredients for consistent mixing, pause the blender every 15 seconds for 1 to 3 minutes at medium-high speed.
- Blend until the consistency you want is achieved. Put one cup of ice in the blender if it's too thin. Add more milk, ¼ cup at a time, if it's too thick.
- Transfer the blend into a bowl and garnish with your preferred toppings, like granola, almonds, seeds, or more fruit.

PER SERVING: Calories: 514; Total fat: 21g; Saturated fat: 3g; Sodium: 139mg; Carbohydrates: 58g; Fiber: 15g; Protein: 28g; Calcium: 452mg; Potassium: 978mg

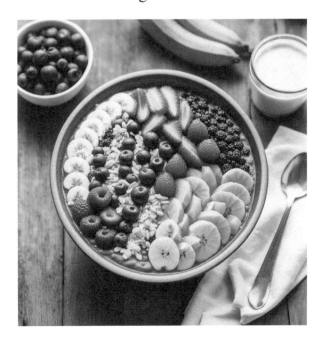

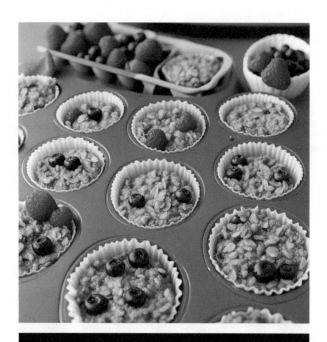

BAKED OATMEAL CUPS

PREP TIME: 10 minutes   COOK TIME: 20 minutes SERVES 6

Ingredients

- Nonstick cooking spray (optional)
- 2 cups rolled oats
- 1 teaspoon baking powder
- 1 teaspoon ground cinnamon, plus more for garnish if desired
- ¼ teaspoon kosher salt
- 1 cup nonfat milk
- 2 large eggs
- ¼ cup maple syrup
- ¼ cup unsweetened applesauce
- 1 teaspoon vanilla extract
- ½ cup dried cranberries
- ½ cup pecan halves

Directions

- Turn the oven on to 350 degrees Fahrenheit. Use cooking spray or paper liners to line a 12-cup muffin pan.
- Combine the oats, baking powder, salt, and cinnamon in a medium-sized bowl.
- Pour in the applesauce, eggs, milk, maple syrup, and vanilla. Mix thoroughly by stirring to blend. Add the pecans and cranberries and fold.
- Evenly distribute the batter among the muffin cups using a ¼-cup measuring scoop. If desired, top each oatmeal cup with cinnamon. A toothpick inserted in the center should come out clean after 20 minutes of baking, or until the tops are golden brown. Give it a few minutes to cool.
- Remaining oatmeal cups can be frozen for up to three months or kept at room temperature for up to five days in an airtight container. Warm in a 350°F oven for 3 to 5 minutes or in a microwave on high for 1 minute, if preferred.

PER SERVING: Calories: 293; Total fat: 10g; Saturated fat: 1g; Sodium: 95mg; Carbohydrates: 44g; Fiber: 5g; Protein: 8g; Calcium: 132mg; Potassium: 347mg

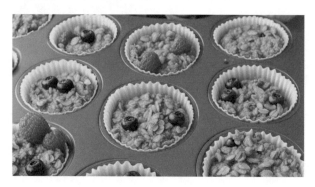

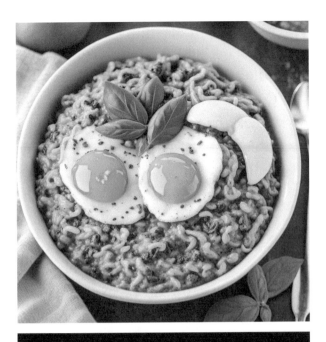

SAVORY PESTO OATS

PREP TIME: 5 minutes   COOK TIME: 5 minutes SERVES 2

Ingredients

- Nonstick cooking spray
- 1 cup rolled oats
- 1¾ cups chicken or vegetable broth
- 2 tablespoons Spinach-Pistachio Pesto Sauce or any store-bought pesto
- 2 tablespoons shredded part-skim mozzarella cheese, plus more for garnish
- 2 large eggs
- Red pepper flakes, for garnish (optional)

Directions

- Apply cooking spray to a nonstick skillet set over medium heat.
- Combine the oats and broth in a bowl that can be placed in the microwave. Three minutes on high in the microwave.
- Take out of the microwave and mix in the mozzarella cheese and pesto. Separate into two bowls.
- Prepare the eggs to your liking (over easy or sunny-side up work great) while the oatmeal is in the microwave. Top each bowl of oats with a cooked egg. Add more mozzarella and, if using, red pepper flakes as garnish.

PER SERVING: Calories: 378; Total fat: 18g; Saturated fat: 5g; Sodium: 451mg; Carbohydrates: 35g; Fiber: 5g; Protein: 17g; Calcium: 147mg; Potassium: 300mg

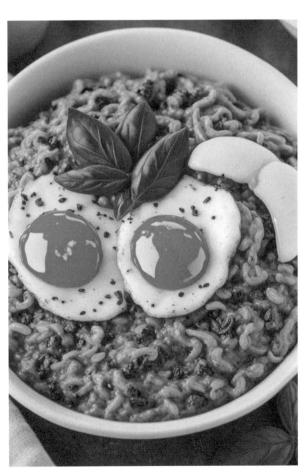

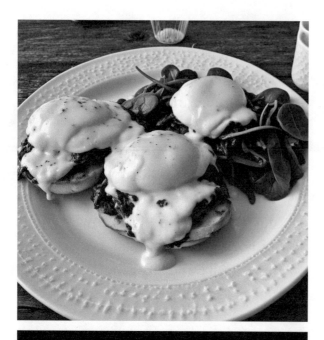

SPINACH AND CHEDDAR ALMOST EGGS BENEDICT

PREP TIME: 5 minutes   COOK TIME: 5 minutes SERVES 2

Ingredients

- 2 whole-grain English muffins, split
- 2 tablespoons olive oil, divided
- 6 cups fresh baby spinach
- 4 large eggs
- 4 slices deli cheddar cheese, such as Vermont cheddar
- Salt
- Freshly ground black pepper

Directions

- Divide the English muffins between two dishes after lightly toasting them.
- Heat 1 tablespoon of oil in a large nonstick skillet over medium heat. Add the spinach and cook for 2 to 3 minutes, or until it just begins to wilt.
- After taking the spinach out of the skillet, distribute it evenly over the English muffins.
- Crack the eggs into the remaining 1 tablespoon of heated oil in the same skillet. Let it cook for one minute, or until the yolks are set and the bottoms are a little browned. Reduce the heat to low, turn the eggs over, and place a piece of cheese on top of each egg. Cook, covered, until the cheese melts, about 1 minute. There will be some runniness in the yolks. Cook for another 1 to 2 minutes if you want a firmer yolk.
- Take the skillet off of the burner after uncovering it. Top the English muffins with spinach and then the eggs and cheese. Add salt and pepper for seasoning, then start enjoying right away.

PER SERVING: Calories: 644; Total fat: 44g; Saturated fat: 16g;
Sodium: 892mg; Carbohydrates: 31g; Fiber: 6g; Protein: 34g;
Calcium: 698mg; Potassium: 822mg

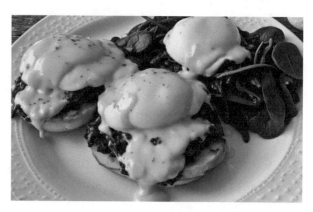

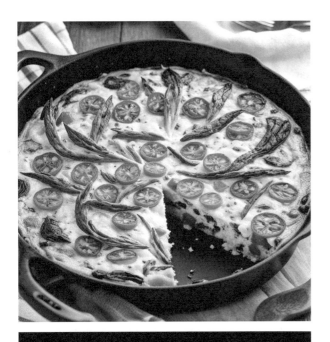

BAKED VEGETABLE FRITTATA

PREP TIME: 5 minutes   COOK TIME: 25 minutes SERVES 6

Ingredients
- Nonstick cooking spray
- 8 large eggs
- 2 tablespoons nonfat milk
- Salt
- Freshly ground black pepper
- 1 cup baby spinach, packed
- ¼ cup grape tomatoes, halved
- ¼ cup shredded cheddar cheese or other cheese of choice, plus more for topping if desired

Directions
- Oven temperature: 400ºF. Apply cooking spray to an 8-by-8-inch baking dish.
- Whisk the milk and eggs together in a medium bowl, then add salt and pepper to taste. Add the cheese, tomatoes, and spinach and stir.
- Fill the baking pan with the mixture. If desired, add a little more cheese on top. Bake until the center is firm, about 20 minutes. After five minutes of cooling, cut into six squares.
- Reheat leftovers in the microwave on high for one minute or store them in the fridge for up to four days.

PER SERVING: Calories: 118; Total fat: 8g; Saturated fat: 3g; Sodium: 157mg; Carbohydrates: 1g; Fiber: 1g; Protein: 10g; Calcium: 81mg; Potassium: 146mg

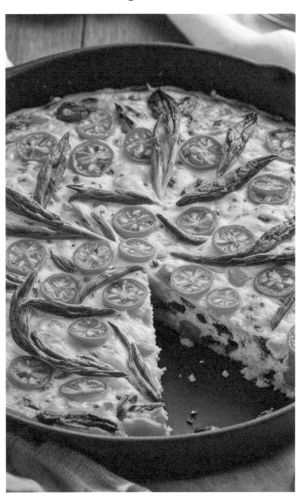

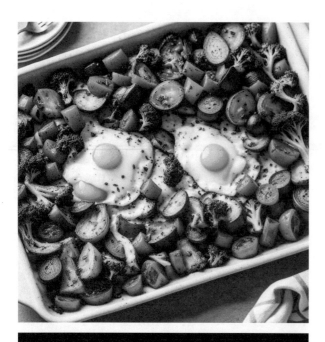

SHEET PAN VEGGIE HASH

PREP TIME: 5 minutes   COOK TIME: 25 minutes SERVES 6

Ingredients

- 2 cups chopped fresh or frozen broccoli florets
- 2 cups sliced mushrooms
- 1 cup diced red onion
- 1 cup diced red bell pepper
- 1 cup grape tomatoes, halved
- 2 tablespoons olive oil
- 1 teaspoon dried thyme
- Salt
- Freshly ground black pepper
- 6 large eggs
- ½ cup shredded cheddar Jack cheese

Directions

- The oven should be preheated to 425°. Use nonstick aluminum foil to line a sheet pan.
- Add the bell pepper, tomatoes, onions, mushrooms, and broccoli to a big bowl. Season with salt and pepper, then add the olive oil and thyme. Coat the vegetables by stirring.
- Arrange the vegetables on the sheet pan in a single layer. Bake for 15 minutes on the center oven rack.
- The pan should be taken out of the oven. Six wells should be made in the hash using the back of a serving spoon. Pour an egg into one of the wells after cracking it into a small bowl or cup. Continue with the remaining eggs. Over the hash, scatter the shredded cheese.
- Put the pan back in the oven and continue cooking until the egg whites are solid and cooked through, about 6 to 10 more minutes. Cook eggs longer for tougher yolks and less for runny eggs. After taking the eggs out of the oven, they will continue to cook. Serve right away.
- Remaining hash can be kept in the fridge for up to four days.

PER SERVING: Calories: 188; Total fat: 13g; Saturated fat: 2g; Sodium: 172mg; Carbohydrates: 8g; Fiber: 4g; Protein: 11g; Calcium: 117mg; Potassium: 397mg

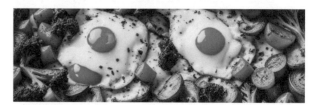

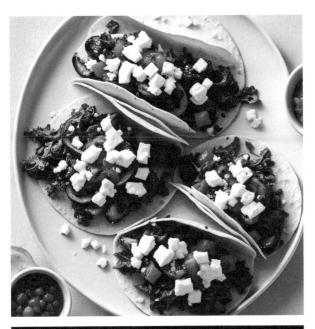

MUSHROOM, KALE, AND FETA BREAKFAST TACOS WITH BRUSCHETTA TOPPNG

PREP TIME: 5 minutes   COOK TIME: 15 minutes SERVES 3

Ingredients

- 1 tablespoon avocado oil
- 1 cup sliced mushrooms
- 4 large eggs
- 1 tablespoon nonfat milk
- ¼ teaspoon dried basil
- ⅛ teaspoon freshly ground black pepper
- 1 cup chopped kale
- Nonstick cooking spray (optional)
- ¼ cup crumbled feta cheese
- 6 (6-inch) corn tortillas
- 1 cup prepared tomato bruschetta topping

Directions

- Heat the oil in a 10-inch skillet over medium heat.
- Add the mushrooms and cook, stirring frequently, until they are tender, 2 to 3 minutes.
- Whisk the eggs, milk, pepper, and basil in a small bowl and set aside.
- After adding the kale to the skillet, cook it for one minute, or until it wilts.
- Before adding the egg mixture to the skillet, if necessary, coat it with cooking spray. Scramble the eggs and vegetables together with a spatula. Add the feta crumbles and continue to sauté until the cheese is melted, about 1 minute after the eggs have set.
- Divide the egg mixture among the tortillas to assemble the tacos, then top each with a bruschetta topping.

PER SERVING: Calories: 293; Total fat: 15g; Saturated fat: 5g; Sodium: 239mg; Carbohydrates: 26g; Fiber: 4g; Protein: 15g; Calcium: 159mg; Potassium: 417mg

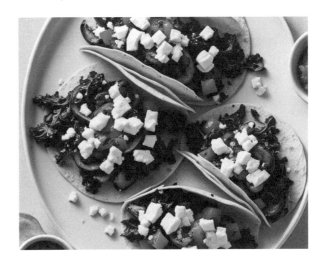

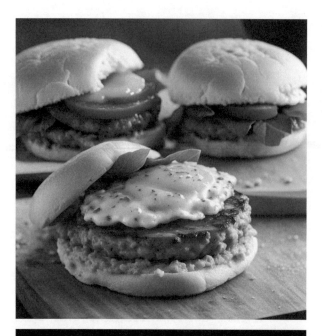

TURKEY SAUSAGE BREAKFAST SANDWICHES

PREP TIME: 10 minutes   COOK TIME: 15 minutes SERVES 6

Ingredients

- 1 pound ground turkey
- 1 teaspoon dried fennel
- 1 teaspoon ground sage
- ½ teaspoon onion powder
- ½ teaspoon garlic powder
- ½ teaspoon dried parsley
- ¼ teaspoon sea salt
- ⅛ teaspoon freshly ground black pepper
- 1 tablespoon olive oil
- 6 whole-wheat English muffins, split
- 6 Granny Smith apple slices, ¼ inch thick
- 6 slices deli cheddar cheese

Directions

- The ground turkey, fennel, sage, onion powder, garlic powder, parsley, salt, and pepper should all be combined in a big basin. Mix the ingredients together with your hands until thoroughly combined.
- Form the turkey into six roughly 3-inch-diameter patties.
- On high, preheat the oven broiler.
- Heat the olive oil in a large ovenproof skillet over medium heat. The sausage patties should be cooked through (internal temperature of 165°F) after 5 minutes on each side.
- Use the toaster to toast the English muffins.
- Remove the patties from the heat and place a slice of apple and a slice of cheddar cheese on top of each one. To melt the cheese, place the pan in the broiler for 60 to 90 seconds.
- Put a patty on either side of an English muffin. Place the other half on top. Serve right away.
- Remaining patties can be frozen for up to three months or kept in the fridge for three to four days.

PER SERVING: Calories: 465; Total fat: 19g; Saturated fat: 7g; Sodium: 563mg; Carbohydrates: 47g; Fiber: 9g; Protein: 28g; Calcium: 389mg; Potassium: 519mg

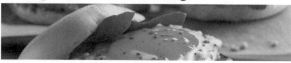

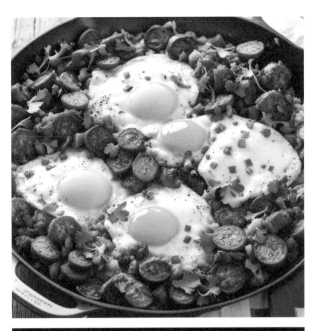

CHICKEN CHORIZO AND EGG BREAKFAST SKILLET

PREP TIME: 5 minutes   COOK TIME: 10 minutes SERVES 4

Ingredients

- 2 tablespoons avocado oil, divided
- 2 chicken chorizo sausage links, diced
- 1 jalapeño, seeds removed and diced (optional)
- 6 large eggs
- ¼ cup scallions, sliced
- 2 tablespoons nonfat milk
- 1 (10-ounce) can fire roasted diced tomatoes with green chiles, drained (or plain diced tomatoes)
- ½ cup shredded four-cheese Mexican blend
- 1 avocado, peeled, pitted, and diced

Directions

- Heat 1 tablespoon of oil in a 10-inch nonstick skillet over medium heat.
- Add the jalapeño (if using) and chorizo, and cook for 5 minutes, or until the jalapeño is soft and the chorizo is browned.
- Whisk the eggs, milk, and scallions together in a small bowl and set aside.
- Add diced tomatoes and chilies and toss until mixed with the chorizo and jalapeño combination. Pour in the egg mixture and the remaining 1 tablespoon of oil.
- Push the mixture to the side of the pan with a rubber spatula to scramble the eggs until curds begin to form. Add the cheese and whisk until melted and mixed in with the solidified eggs. Take off the heat and sprinkle the diced avocado on top. Serve right away.
- You can keep leftovers in the fridge for up to four days.

PER SERVING: Calories: 442; Total fat: 35g; Saturated fat: 10g; Sodium: 678mg; Carbohydrates: 9g; Fiber: 5g; Protein: 22g; Calcium: 183mg; Potassium: 593mg

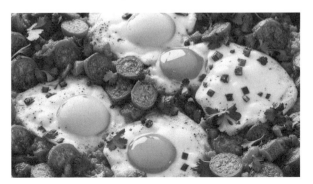

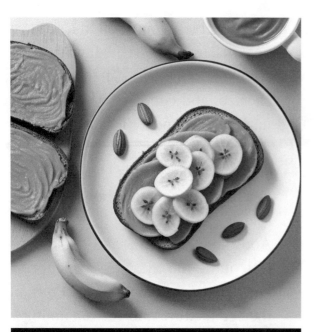

SWEET POTATO TOAST WITH ALMOND BUTTER AND BANANA

PREP TIME: 5 minutes   COOK TIME: 15 minutes SERVES 4

Ingredients

- 1 large (or 2 medium) sweet potatoes, unpeeled, cut diagonally into ¼ -inch slices
- Nonstick cooking spray
- 2 tablespoons almond butter (or any nut or seed butter)
- 1 banana, sliced
- Hemp seeds, for garnish
- Cinnamon, for garnish
- Honey, for garnish

Directions

- Apply cooking spray to the sweet potato slices on both sides. Toast the slices on the highest setting while placing them directly on the toaster oven rack. Continue toasting until the

- sweet potato slices are cooked through, have a toasted and browned outside, and are starting to get a little crisp. This could take two or three rounds, with each round lasting roughly five minutes. It can take a little longer to cook if you use a pop-up toaster.
- Place a few banana slices on top of the potato slices after spreading almond butter on them. Add hemp seeds, cinnamon, and honey as garnish.

PER SERVING: Calories: 109; Total fat: 5g; Saturated fat: 0g; Sodium: 19mg; Carbohydrates: 15g; Fiber: 3g; Protein: 3g; Calcium: 39mg; Potassium: 275mg

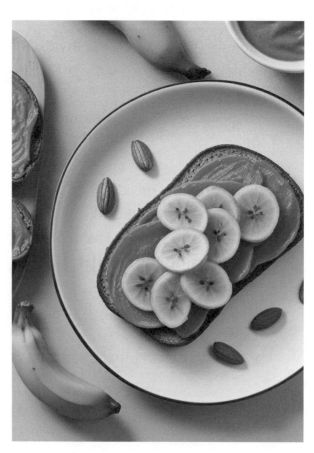

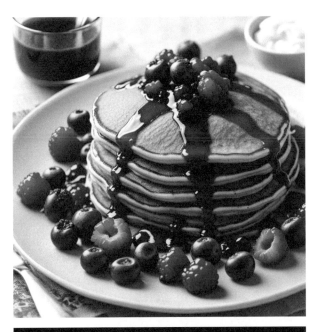

BUCKWHEAT PANCAKES WITH BERRY COMPOTE

PREP TIME: 5 minutes   COOK TIME: 25 minutes SERVES 4

Ingredients

- 2 cups frozen mixed berries
- 2 tablespoons pomegranate juice
- ¾ cup buckwheat flour
- ¾ cup self-rising flour (see Simple Swap)
- 1 tablespoon sugar
- ¼ teaspoon baking soda
- ½ teaspoon ground cinnamon
- 2 teaspoons chia seeds, divided
- 2 large eggs
- 1 cup buttermilk
- 1 teaspoon vanilla extract
- 2 tablespoons canola oil
- ½ cup water
- Nonstick cooking spray

Directions

- Combine the pomegranate juice and frozen berries in a small saucepan over medium heat. Reduce the heat to low and simmer the compote uncovered for 10 minutes, stirring regularly, when it starts to boil.
- Buckwheat flour, self-rising flour, sugar, baking soda, cinnamon, and 1 teaspoon of chia seeds should all be combined in a big basin. Combine.
- Whisk the eggs, buttermilk, water, oil, and vanilla extract in a medium-sized bowl.
- Pour the egg and buttermilk combination into the well created in the middle of the dry ingredients. Mix until incorporated.
- Apply cooking spray to a nonstick pan or griddle and place it over medium-high heat. Fill each pancake with ¼ cup of batter. Cook until little bubbles appear in the batter, 2 to 3 minutes on one side, then turn and cook for another 1 to 2 minutes.
- Remove the berry compote from the heat and add the remaining 1 teaspoon of chia seeds after it is ready. Let it cool.
- Top pancakes with warm berry compote and serve.
- Keep any leftover pancakes in the fridge for up to three days and any leftover compote for up to a week.

PER SERVING: Calories: 354; Total fat: 12g; Saturated fat: 2g; Sodium:

- 518mg; Carbohydrates: 52g; Fiber: 6g; Protein: 11g; Calcium:
- 202mg; Potassium: 359mg

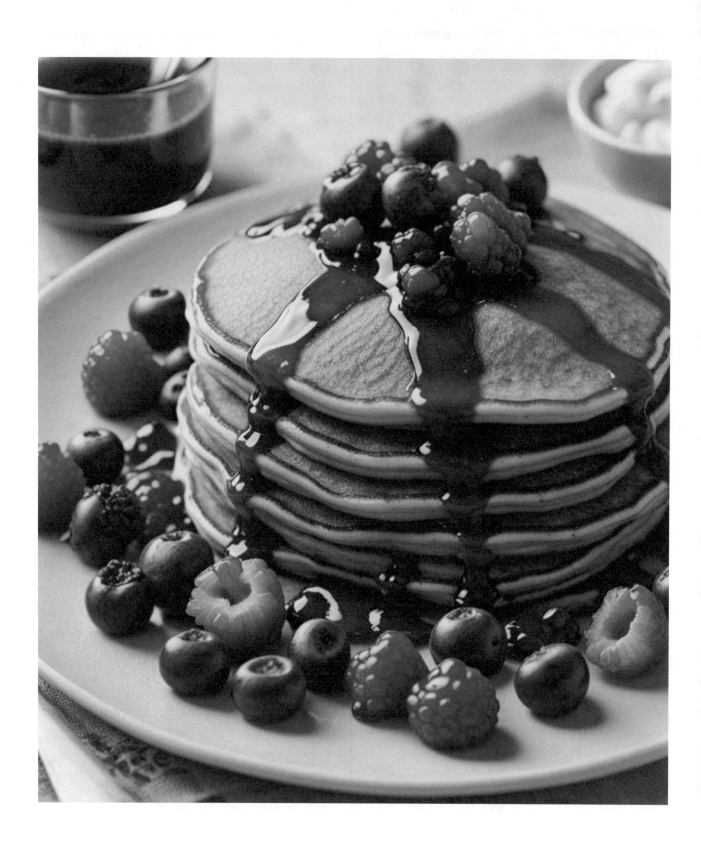

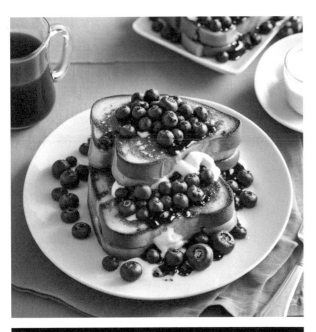

BLUEBERRY-RICOTTA-STUFFED FRENCH TOAST

PREP TIME: 5 minutes   COOK TIME: 15 minutes SERVES 4

Ingredients

- 6 large eggs
- ¼ cup nonfat milk
- ¼ teaspoon vanilla extract
- ¼ teaspoon ground cinnamon
- 1 tablespoon butter or nonstick cooking spray
- 1 loaf brioche or challah bread, cut into 1-inch slices
- 1 cup part-skim ricotta cheese
- 1 cup fresh or defrosted frozen blueberries, divided

Directions

- Whisk the eggs, milk, cinnamon, and vanilla in a medium basin. Put aside.

- Grease a nonstick pan or griddle with cooking spray or butter and preheat it over medium-high heat.
- Place the bread slices on the griddle and cook for 3 to 5 minutes on each side, or until browned, after dipping them into the egg mixture to coat them on both sides.
- The ricotta should be placed in a small bowl. Puree ¼ cup of blueberries in a food processor or blender. Stir in the remaining ¾ cup of blueberries after folding the blueberry puree into the ricotta cheese. Refrigerate, covered, until ready to use.
- After removing the bread from the griddle, cover one slice with ¼ cup of the ricotta filling and cover it with another slice. Serve right away.
- French toast leftovers can be frozen for up to three months or kept in the fridge for up to two days. The filling can be refrigerated for up to two or three days. When serving, warm the bread and top with the ricotta; store the filling and French toast separately.

PER SERVING: Calories: 476; Total fat: 17g; Saturated fat: 8g; Sodium: 711mg; Carbohydrates: 53g; Fiber: 3g; Protein: 26g; Calcium: 280mg; Potassium: 330mg

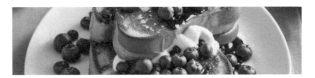

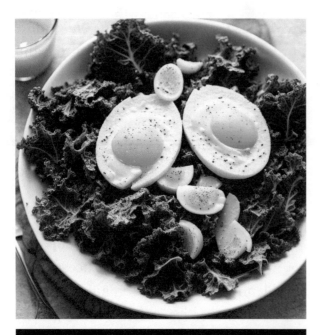

KALE CAESAR SALAD

PREP TIME: 5 minutes   COOK TIME: 10 minutes SERVES 2

Ingredients

- 2 large eggs
- 1 (10-ounce) bag washed, chopped kale
- 2 tablespoons extra-virgin olive oil
- Juice of 1 lemon
- ¼ cup nutritional yeast, plus more for sprinkling if desired
- 2 tablespoons raw, shelled sunflower seeds
- Kosher salt
- Freshly ground black pepper

Directions

- Heat water in a medium pot until it boils. Separate the eggs from one another and carefully drop them into the water using a big slotted spoon. Depending on how done you want the yolk, boil for 6 to 8 minutes after lowering the heat to a low simmer. In a small dish, prepare an ice bath and set it aside.
- Combine the sunflower seeds, nutritional yeast, lemon juice, olive oil, and kale in a big bowl. Add salt and pepper for seasoning. To soften the leaves and mix the kale with the seasonings, knead it with your hands.
- The kale greens should be split between two plates. If desired, sprinkle more nutritional yeast on top.
- For one minute, move the eggs into the ice bath using the slotted spoon. Place the soft-boiled eggs on top of the kale greens after carefully removing the shells under cold running water. Add more salt and pepper to taste and serve right away.

PER SERVING: Calories: 347; Total fat: 24g; Saturated fat: 4g; Sodium: 216mg; Carbohydrates: 18g; Fiber: 7g; Protein: 18g; Calcium: 252mg; Potassium: 978mg

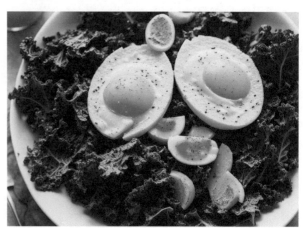

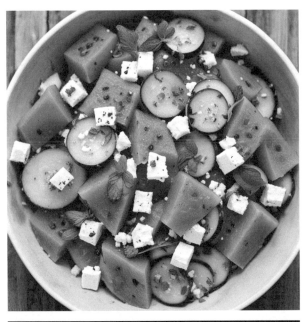

WATERMELON, TOMATO, CUCUMBER, FETA, AND MINT SALAD

PREP TIME: 5 minutes SERVES 4

Ingredients

- 4 cups seedless watermelon, cubed
- 3 cups red or yellow grape tomatoes, halved
- ½ seedless English cucumber, sliced
- 1 (8-ounce) block feta cheese, diced
- ¼ cup fresh mint leaves, sliced
- Balsamic glaze, for topping
- Sea salt (optional)
- Freshly ground black pepper (optional)

Directions

- Combine the watermelon, cucumbers, tomatoes, feta cheese, and mint in a big bowl.
- The mixture should be divided among four plates. Pour balsamic glaze over it. If used, season with sea salt and pepper.

PER SERVING: Calories: 225; Total fat: 13g; Saturated fat: 9g; Sodium: 529mg; Carbohydrates: 20g; Fiber: 2g; Protein: 10g; Calcium: 309mg; Potassium: 532mg

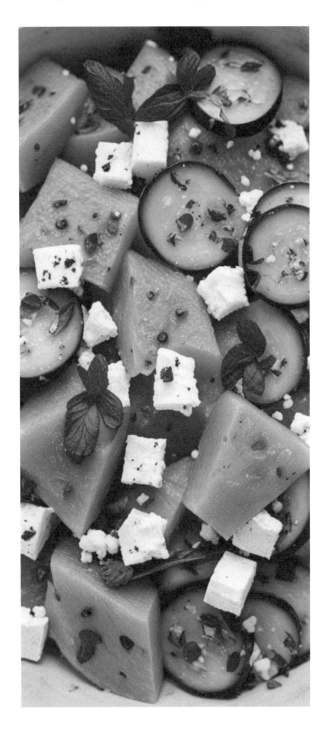

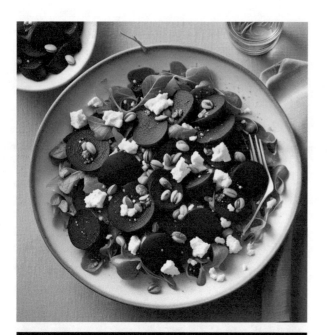

BEET, GOAT CHEESE, AND PISTACHIO SALAD

PREP TIME: 5 minutes SERVES 4

Ingredients

- 4 cups mixed greens
- 1 (6.5-ounce) package cooked beets, quartered
- ¼ cup crumbled goat cheese
- 2 tablespoons chopped shelled pistachios
- ½ cup Lemon-Shallot Champagne Vinaigrette or any store-bought lemon vinaigrette

Directions

- The mixed greens should be divided among four plates. Add the goat cheese and beets on top, then the chopped pistachios. Pour the vinaigrette over it.

PER SERVING: Calories: 138; Total fat: 10g; Saturated fat: 2g; Sodium: 363mg; Carbohydrates: 10g; Fiber: 2g; Protein: 4g; Calcium: 44mg; Potassium: 337mg

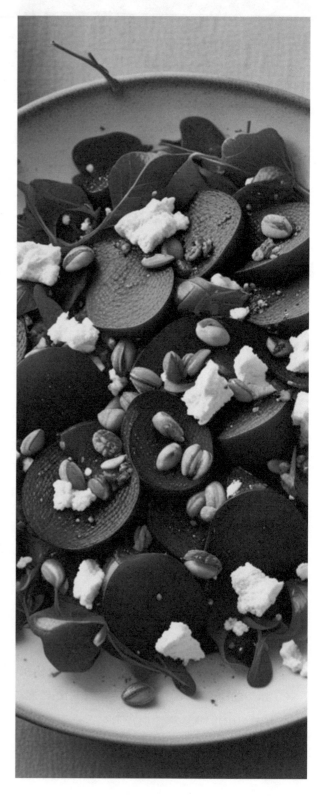

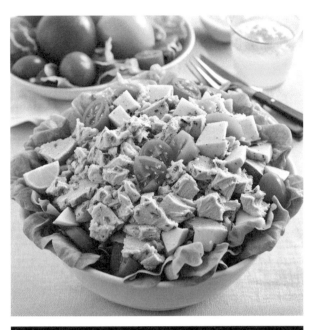

TANGY NO-MAYO TUNA SALAD

PREP TIME: 10 minutes SERVES 6

Ingredients

- 2 (12-ounce) cans albacore tuna in water, drained
- ½ cup chopped mini sweet bell peppers
- ¼ cup diced celery
- 2 tablespoons pitted, sliced Kalamata olives
- 2 tablespoons white wine vinegar
- Juice of 1 lemon
- 1 tablespoon extra-virgin olive oil
- ½ teaspoon freshly ground black pepper
- ¼ teaspoon kosher salt

Directions

- Put the tuna, peppers, celery, olives, vinegar, lemon juice, olive oil, salt, and pepper in a big bowl. Combine
- all the ingredients with a fork.
- Tuna salad leftovers can be kept in the fridge for up to five days.

PER SERVING: Calories: 112; Total fat: 4g; Saturated fat: 1g; Sodium: 310mg; Carbohydrates: 2g; Fiber: 0g; Protein: 19g; Calcium: 22mg; Potassium: 217mg

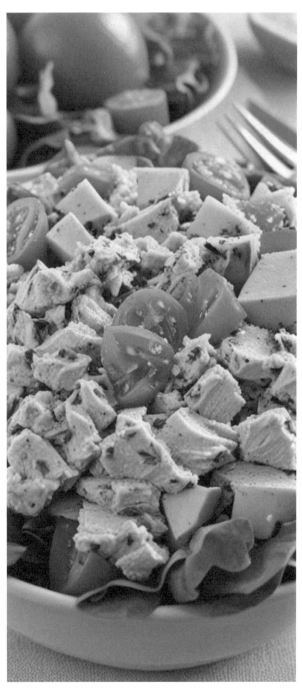

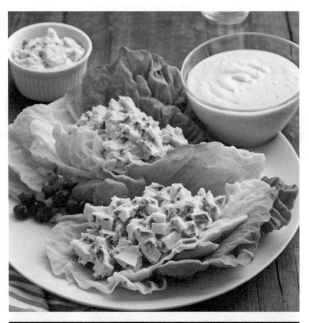

WALDORF CHICKEN SALAD LETTUCE WRAPS

PREP TIME: 20 minutes SERVES 6

Ingredients
- 2 cups chopped cooked chicken
- ½ red apple (such as Honeycrisp), diced
- ½ cup red seedless grapes, halved
- ½ cup diced celery
- ½ cup chopped walnuts
- ½ cup plain nonfat Greek yogurt
- ¼ cup olive oil mayonnaise
- 1 teaspoon dried tarragon
- ⅛ teaspoon salt
- ⅛ teaspoon freshly ground black pepper
- 1 head Bibb lettuce

Directions
- Put the walnuts, celery, apples, grapes, and chicken in a big bowl.
- Whisk the yogurt, mayonnaise, tarragon, salt, and pepper in a small bowl. Stir to coat after adding to the chicken salad mixture.
- To make wraps, serve the chicken salad with Bibb lettuce leaves.
- Any leftover chicken salad can be kept in the fridge for up to five days in an airtight container.

PER SERVING: Calories: 205; Total fat: 12g; Saturated fat: 2g; Sodium: 168mg; Carbohydrates: 8g; Fiber: 2g; Protein: 17g; Calcium: 53mg; Potassium: 315mg

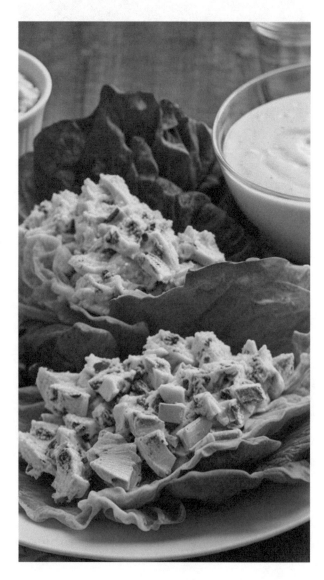

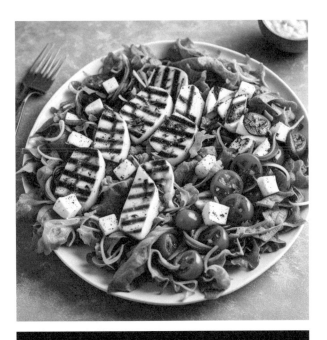

GRILLED HALLOUMI SALAD

PREP TIME: 10 minutes   **COOK TIME: 5 minutes SERVES 4**

Ingredients

- Nonstick cooking spray
- 8 ounces Halloumi cheese, cut into ½ -inch slices
- 2 cups mixed greens
- ½ red apple (such as Honeycrisp), thinly sliced
- ¼ cup pecan halves
- ¼ cup pomegranate arils
- ½ cup Lemon-Shallot Champagne Vinaigrette or any store-bought vinaigrette

Directions

- Heat a 10-inch nonstick skillet or grill pan to a medium-high temperature. Apply cooking spray. After placing the halloumi slices on the pan, fry them for three minutes on each side, or until they are tender and gently browned.
- The mixed greens should be divided among four bowls. Place the pomegranate arils, pecans, and apple slices on top. Place the grilled halloumi on top, then pour the vinaigrette over it.

PER SERVING: Calories: 291; Total fat: 23g; Saturated fat: 10g;
Sodium: 431mg; Carbohydrates: 13g;
Fiber: 2g; Protein: 9g;
Calcium: 300mg; Potassium: 204mg

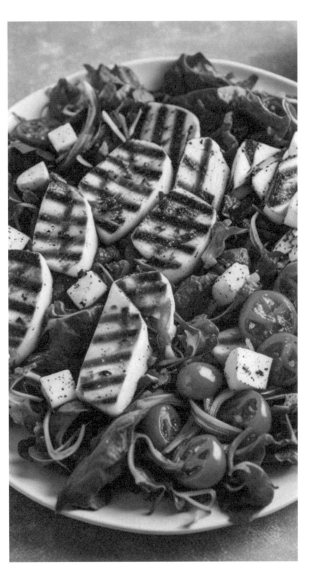

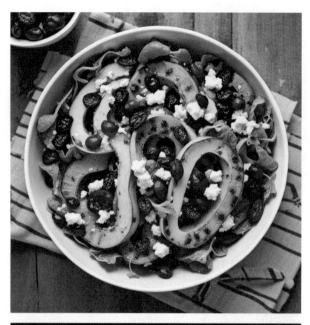

ROASTED DELICATA SQUASH, CRANBERRY, AND GORGONZOLA SALAD

PREP TIME: 5 minutes   COOK TIME: 20 minutes SERVES 4

Ingredients

- 1 large delicata squash
- 1 tablespoon olive oil
- 1 tablespoon honey
- ½ teaspoon dried thyme
- Salt
- Freshly ground black pepper
- 4 cups arugula
- ¼ cup dried cranberries
- ¼ cup unsalted pepitas
- ¼ cup Gorgonzola cheese
- ½ cup Raspberry–Poppy Seed Dressing

Directions

- Prepare a sheet pan with nonstick aluminum foil and preheat the oven to 425ºF.
- Cut the squash in half lengthwise after slicing off the ends. Scoop out the seeds with a spoon. Cut the halves into ¼-inch slices after placing them flat-sides down.
- Put the squash, honey, thyme, and olive oil in a zip-top bag and shake to coat. After taking the squash out of the bag, arrange it on the sheet pan in a single layer, sprinkle it with salt and pepper, and roast it for 20 minutes, rotating it midway through.
- Arrange the arugula in four bowls and garnish with the Gorgonzola, pepitas, and dried cranberries. Drizzle the dressing over the cooked squash.
- Salad leftovers without dressing can be kept in the fridge for up to two days.

PER SERVING: Calories: 220; Total fat: 12g; Saturated fat: 3g; Sodium: 431mg; Carbohydrates: 27g; Fiber: 3g; Protein: 5g; Calcium: 122mg; Potassium: 561mg

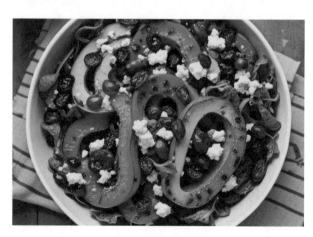

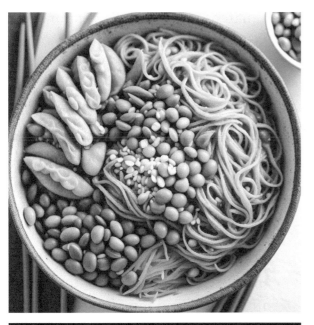

COLD SESAME NOODLE BOWL

PREP TIME: 5 minutes   COOK TIME: 5 minutes SERVES 4

Ingredients

- 1 (10-ounce package) udon or soba noodles
- ½ cup Sesame, Miso, and Ginger Dressing or store-bought dressing
- 1 cup frozen shelled edamame, thawed
- ¼ cup scallions, thinly sliced
- 2 tablespoons sesame seeds, toasted (see Technique Trick)

Directions

- As directed on the package, bring a saucepan of water to a boil and cook the noodles. Rinse with cold water after draining.
- Put the noodles back in the pot. Coat by adding the dressing and .
- stirring. To combine the noodles and dressing, add the edamame, sesame seeds, and scallions. If necessary, add more dressing. Transfer to bowls, garnish with more ingredients if preferred, and serve.
- You may keep leftover noodles in the fridge for up to five days

PER SERVING: Calories: 383; Total fat: 11g; Saturated fat: 2g; Sodium: 631mg; Carbohydrates: 61g; Fiber: 3g; Protein: 15g; Calcium: 60mg; Potassium: 404mg

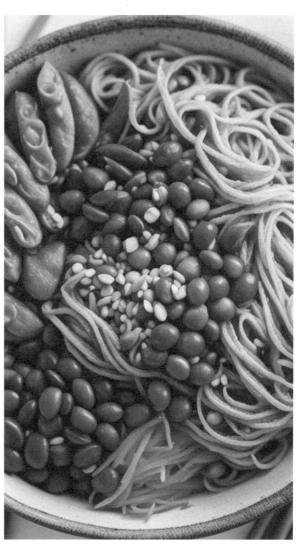

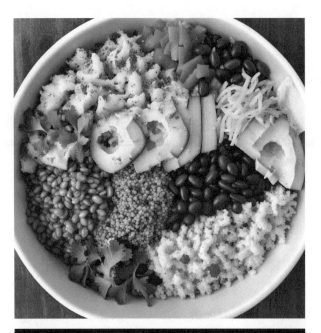

CAULIFLOWER RICE BURRITO BOWL

PREP TIME: 5 minutes   COOK TIME: 10 minutes SERVES 2

Ingredients

- 1 (15.5-ounce) can black beans, drained and rinsed
- 1 cup frozen corn
- 1 (14.5-ounce) can diced tomatoes, drained with juices reserved
- ½ teaspoon chili powder
- ½ teaspoon cumin
- 1 tablespoon avocado oil
- 1 (12-ounce) bag cauliflower rice
- ¼ teaspoon kosher salt
- ¼ cup chopped cilantro, plus more for sprinkling if desired
- Juice of 1 lime
- ¼ cup shredded cheddar Jack cheese

Directions

- Put the beans, frozen corn,

tomatoes, chili powder, cumin, and 2 tablespoons of the tomato juice that was set aside in a small skillet over medium heat. Cook, stirring occasionally, until thoroughly cooked, 3 to 5 minutes.
- Heat the avocado oil in a large nonstick skillet over medium heat. Add the salt and cauliflower rice. Stirring occasionally, sauté for 3 to 5 minutes, or until cooked through and just beginning to soften. Take off the heat and mix in the lime juice and cilantro.
- Place the bean mixture and shredded cheese on top of the cauliflower rice that has been divided between two dishes. If desired, top with chopped cilantro or other ingredients.

PER SERVING: Calories: 461; Total fat: 14g; Saturated fat: 4g; Sodium: 558mg; Carbohydrates: 71g; Fiber: 22g; Protein: 23g; Calcium: 302mg; Potassium: 1,815mg

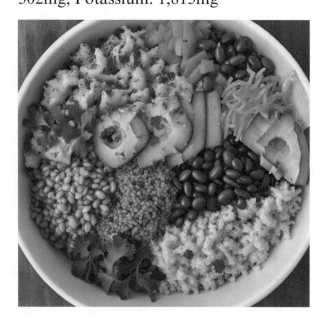

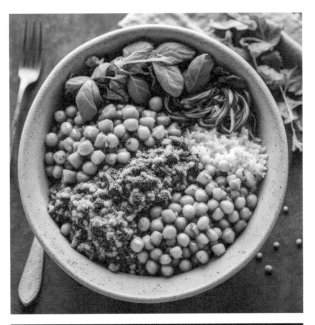

PESTO GRAIN BOWL WITH CHICKPEAS

PREP TIME: 5 minutes   COOK TIME: 15 minutes SERVES 4

Ingredients

- 1 cup uncooked quinoa
- 1½ cups chicken or vegetable broth
- 1 large zucchini, diced
- 1 cup grape tomatoes, halved
- 1 (15.5-ounce) can chickpeas, drained and rinsed
- 1 (8-ounce) container small pearl-size mozzarella balls, drained
- ¼ cup Spinach-Pistachio Pesto Sauce or any store-bought pesto sauce, plus 2 tablespoons

Directions

- As directed on the package, cook the quinoa in the broth.
- Put the chickpeas, tomatoes, zucchini, and mozzarella balls in a big bowl. Add ¼ cup of pesto sauce and stir to coat.
- Stir the remaining 2 tablespoons of pesto sauce into the cooked quinoa.
- After dividing the quinoa among four bowls, add the mozzarella, chickpeas, and veggie combination over top.
- Any remaining grain bowl can be kept for up to three days in the fridge.

PER SERVING: Calories: 560; Total fat: 30g; Saturated fat: 10g; Sodium: 741mg; Carbohydrates: 47g; Fiber: 8g; Protein: 27g; Calcium: 408mg; Potassium: 703mg

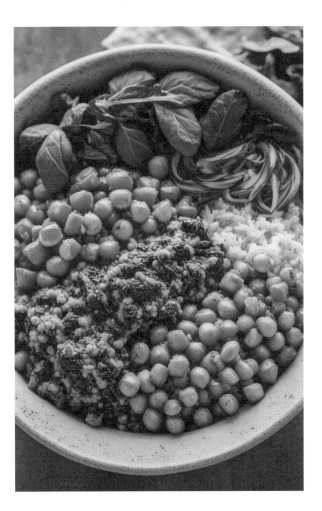

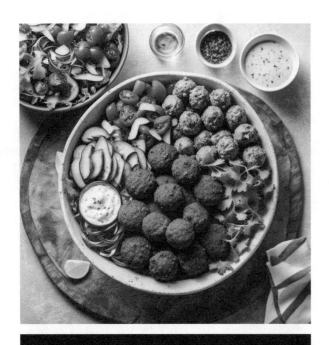

FALAFEL BOWL

PREP TIME: 10 minutes   COOK TIME: 15 minutes SERVES 6

Ingredients

- 2 (15.5-ounce) cans chickpeas, drained and rinsed
- 2 garlic cloves
- ¼ cup fresh parsley
- ¼ cup fresh cilantro
- 1 teaspoon cumin
- ½ teaspoon salt
- ½ teaspoon freshly ground black pepper
- ¼ cup panko bread crumbs
- 1 to 2 tablespoons water
- Nonstick cooking spray
- 6 cups chopped romaine lettuce
- ¾ cup Tzatziki Sauce or store-bought tzatziki sauce

Directions

- Add the chickpeas, cumin, cilantro, garlic, parsley, salt, and pepper to a food processor. Scrape down the sides and pulse a couple times to blend. Pulse one more to mix in the panko. If the dough is too crumbly and dry, add the water.
- Using your hands, form two tablespoon-sized balls. Put the falafel in the basket of the air fryer, spray it with cooking spray, and cook it at 400 degrees Fahrenheit for 15 minutes, turning it halfway through, until it is golden.
- The romaine should be divided among six bowls. Drizzle tzatziki sauce over each bowl after adding three falafels and any extra toppings you like.
- Falafel leftovers can be kept in the fridge for up to five days. For up to three days, keep the romaine in the fridge without dressing.

PER SERVING: Calories: 127; Total fat: 3g; Saturated fat: 0g; Sodium: 366mg; Carbohydrates: 20g; Fiber: 6g; Protein: 7g; Calcium: 72mg; Potassium: 265mg

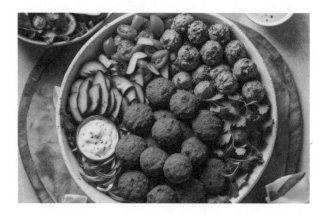

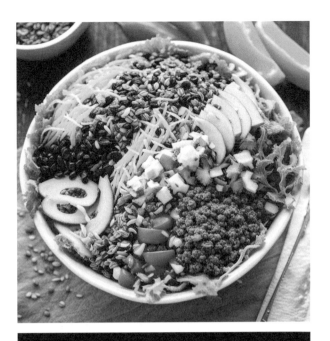

SUNFLOWER TACO SALAD BOWL

PREP TIME: 15 minutes SERVES 4

Ingredients

- 1 cup raw, shelled sunflower seeds
- 2 tablespoons taco seasoning
- 4 cups chopped romaine lettuce
- 1 cup shredded red cabbage
- 1 avocado, peeled, pitted, and diced
- 1 cup diced Oaxaca cheese or shredded four-cheese Mexican blend
- ½ cup fresh refrigerated salsa or pico de gallo
- ½ cup Avocado Buttermilk Ranch Dressing or store-bought Greek yogurt–based ranch dressing (such as Bolthouse Farms)

Directions

- Soak the sunflower seeds for ten minutes in a small dish of water. After draining, combine the seeds and taco seasoning in a blender or food processor. Pulse until well blended and crumbly, similar to ground meat.
- The romaine lettuce should be divided among four dishes. Add the shredded cabbage, avocado, cheese, salsa, ranch dressing, and sunflower taco meat on top.
- Any leftover meat from sunflower tacos can be kept in the fridge for up to five days.

PER SERVING: Calories: 429; Total fat: 32g; Saturated fat: 7g; Sodium: 632mg; Carbohydrates: 24g; Fiber: 9g; Protein: 15g; Calcium: 256mg; Potassium: 770mg

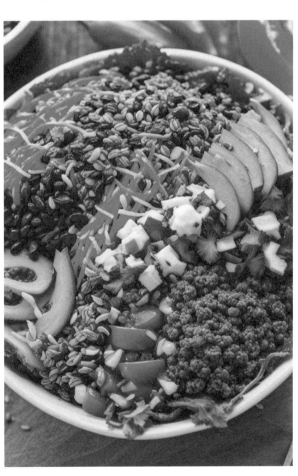

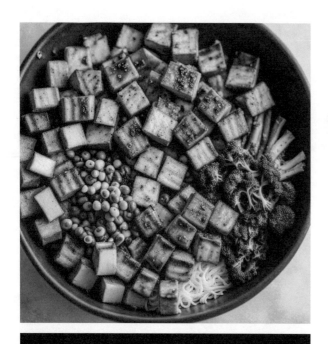

CRISPY TOFU BOWL

PREP TIME: 10 minutes   COOK TIME: 15 minutes SERVES 4

Ingredients

- 1 cup uncooked jasmine rice
- 1 (14-ounce) block extra-firm tofu, drained
- 2 tablespoons low-sodium soy sauce
- 1 tablespoon white miso
- 1 tablespoon sesame oil
- Nonstick cooking spray
- 1 cup shredded carrots
- 1 cup thinly sliced mini sweet bell peppers
- 1 cup shredded red cabbage
- ¼ cup sliced scallions
- ½ cup Sesame, Miso, and Ginger Dressing

Directions

- As directed on the package, cook the rice and set aside.
- To drain the excess liquid, wrap the tofu in layers of paper towels and press. Put a heavy-bottomed saucepan on top to keep the liquid from escaping.
- Mix the miso, sesame oil, and soy sauce in a big basin and whisk until smooth.
- Toss the tofu in the big basin to coat it with the sauce after cutting it into 1-inch cubes.
- Tofu should be layered in the basket of the air fryer, sprayed with cooking spray, and cooked at 400°F for 15 minutes, tossing halfway through.
- Place the bell peppers, cabbage, scallions, and carrots on top of the rice, which has been divided among four bowls. Drizzle the dressing over the tofu.
- Remaining bowls can be kept in the fridge for up to a day.

PER SERVING: Calories: 404; Total fat: 16g; Saturated fat: 2g; Sodium: 541mg; Carbohydrates: 51g; Fiber: 3g; Protein: 15g; Calcium: 240mg; Potassium: 478mg

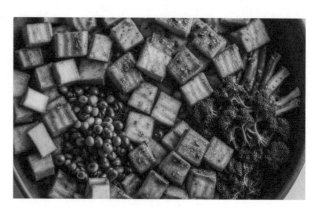

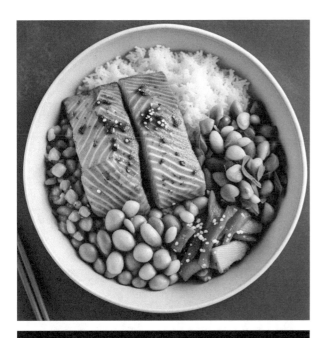

SALMON TERIYAKI POWER BOWL

PREP TIME: 5 minutes   COOK TIME: 10 minutes SERVES 4

Ingredients

- 2 (8-ounce) packages precooked brown rice
- 4 (4-ounce) skinless salmon fillets
- ¾ cup teriyaki sauce, divided, plus more for drizzling
- 1 pound sliced shiitake or cremini mushrooms
- 1 cup frozen shelled edamame, thawed
- 1 cup shredded red cabbage
- ⅔ cup shredded carrots
- 2 tablespoons sliced scallions (optional)

Directions

- Line a sheet pan with nonstick aluminum foil and preheat the oven broiler to high.
- As directed on the package, microwave the brown rice and set aside.
- Combine the salmon and half a cup of teriyaki sauce in a big bowl or zip-top bag.
- Combine the mushrooms and the remaining ¼ cup of teriyaki sauce in a another small bowl or bag.
- Set aside the leftover sauce and place the salmon on the lined sheet pan. For three minutes, broil the fish. Take the salmon out of the broiler, turn it over, drizzle it with the teriyaki sauce you set up, place the mushrooms on top, and continue to broil it for two more minutes.
- Divide the rice, carrots, cabbage, and edamame across four bowls. Place the mushrooms and grilled fish on top. Top with the scallions, if using. If desired, drizzle with more teriyaki sauce.
- Keep any leftover salmon apart from the vegetables and rice. For three to five minutes, reheat the salmon in the oven or under the broiler. Serve the rice and veggies cold or reheat in the microwave for 1 to 2 minutes.

PER SERVING: Calories: 441; Total fat: 10g; Saturated fat: 2g; Sodium: 716mg; Carbohydrates: 50g; Fiber: 8g; Protein: 38g; Calcium: 108mg; Potassium: 1,317mg

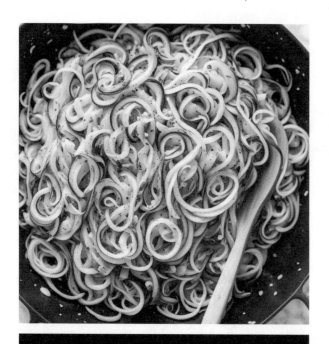

SPICY GARLICKY ZOODLES

PREP TIME: 5 minutes   COOK TIME: 5 minutes SERVES 4

Ingredients

- 1 tablespoon olive oil
- 4 garlic cloves, minced
- 1 teaspoon red pepper flakes
- 1 pound zucchini, spiralized
- ¼ teaspoon salt
- Grated Parmesan cheese, for garnish (optional)

Directions

- Heat the oil in a large nonstick skillet over medium heat. Sauté the red pepper flakes and garlic for about 30 seconds, or until aromatic.
- Add the zoodles, garlic, and red pepper flakes, and cook for 4 minutes, or until the zoodles are tender.
- Add salt to the zoodles and, if using,

- sprinkle some Parmesan cheese on top.
- Remaining cooked zoodles can be kept in the fridge for up to two days

PER SERVING: Calories: 54; Total fat: 4g; Saturated fat: 1g; Sodium: 155mg; Carbohydrates: 5g; Fiber: 1g; Protein: 2g; Calcium: 24mg; Potassium: 308mg

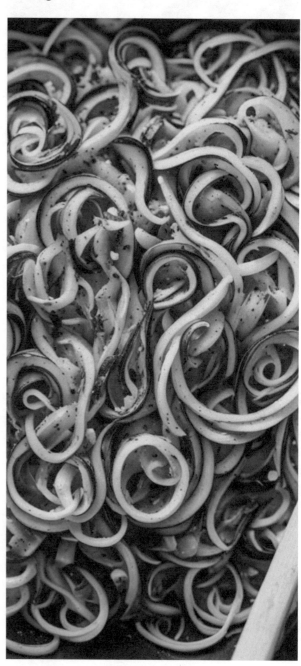

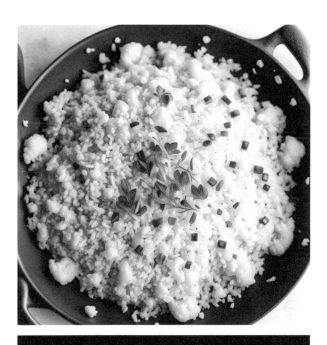

CAULIFLOWER RISOTTO

PREP TIME: 5 minutes   COOK TIME: 15 minutes SERVES 2

Ingredients

- 2 tablespoons olive oil
- 2 garlic cloves, minced
- 1 (12-ounce) package fresh cauliflower rice (about 2 cups)
- 1 cup vegetable stock or broth
- 1 cup shredded or grated Parmesan cheese
- 1 teaspoon dried thyme

Directions

- Heat the oil in a medium nonstick skillet over medium heat. Sauté the garlic for one to two minutes, or until it becomes transparent.
- Add the broth after stirring the cauliflower to coat it with oil. Simmer for 10 minutes, stirring now and again, until the liquid is absorbed.
- After taking the skillet off of the burner, add the thyme and Parmesan cheese and stir. Serve right away.
- Remaining risotto can be kept in the fridge for up to two days.

PER SERVING: Calories: 383; Total fat: 28g; Saturated fat: 10g; Sodium: 932mg; Carbohydrates: 18g; Fiber: 4g; Protein: 17g; Calcium: 471mg; Potassium: 613mg

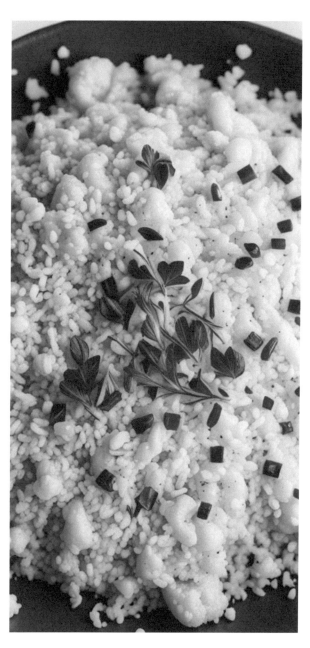

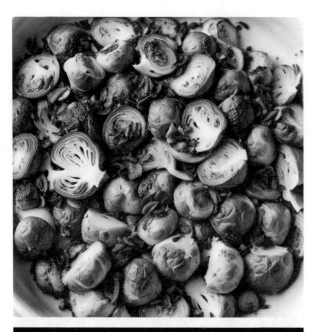

ROASTED SHAVED BRUSSELS SPROUTS

PREP TIME: 5 minutes   COOK TIME: 15 minutes SERVES 2

Ingredients

- 1 pound Brussels sprouts, shaved
- ¼ cup olive oil
- ½ teaspoon salt, plus more for seasoning
- ½ teaspoon freshly ground black pepper, plus more for seasoning
- Parmesan cheese, for garnish (optional)

Directions

- Set the oven temperature to 450 degrees Fahrenheit. Use nonstick aluminum foil or parchment paper to line a sheet pan.
- Combine the shaved Brussels sprouts, salt, pepper, and olive oil in a big bowl. On the prepared sheet

pan, arrange them in a single layer. If necessary, add more salt and pepper for seasoning.
- The Brussels sprouts should be crisp and caramelized after 15 minutes of roasting. After taking them out of the oven, top them with Parmesan cheese, if using.
- Any leftover Brussels sprouts can be kept for up to three days in the fridge. To re-crisp, reheat in an oven set to 350ºF for 5 minutes.

PER SERVING: Calories: 336; Total fat: 28g; Saturated fat: 4g; Sodium: 639mg; Carbohydrates: 20g; Fiber: 9g; Protein: 8g; Calcium: 96mg; Potassium: 886mg

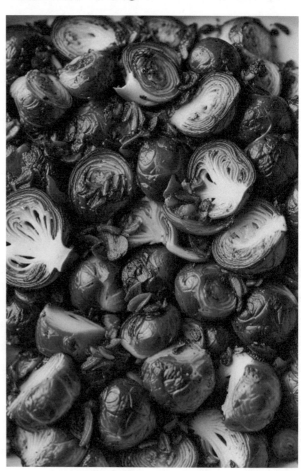

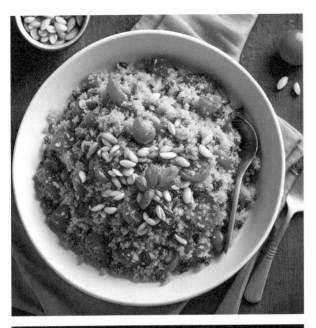

QUINOA WITH TOASTED PINE NUTS AND TOMATOE

PREP TIME: 5 minutes   COOK TIME: 25 minutes SERVES 4

Ingredients

- ¼ cup pine nuts
- 2 tablespoons olive oil
- ½ sweet onion, diced
- 1 cup uncooked quinoa
- 1½ cups low-sodium chicken broth
- ½ cup halved grape tomatoes
- ¼ cup chopped fresh parsley
- Juice of ½ lemon

Directions

- Toast the pine nuts in an ungreased medium saucepan over medium heat, turning constantly until aromatic and toasted, 30 seconds. After taking the pine nuts out of the pan, place them aside.
- Fill the pot with the olive oil. Add the onions and cook for 3 minutes, or until they are transparent.
- To toast, add the quinoa and cook it for two minutes with the onions.
- Bring the mixture to a boil, add the broth, cover, and lower the heat to low. Simmer until nearly all of the liquid has been absorbed, 10 to 12 minutes.
- After turning off the heat, leave the pot covered for five minutes to allow the liquid to completely soak.
- Add the lemon juice, parsley, tomatoes, and pine nuts and stir. Serve right away.
- Keep leftovers in the fridge for up to two or three days.

PER SERVING: Calories: 279; Total fat: 15g; Saturated fat: 2g; Sodium: 46mg; Carbohydrates: 30g; Fiber: 4g; Protein: 7g; Calcium: 29mg; Potassium: 361mg

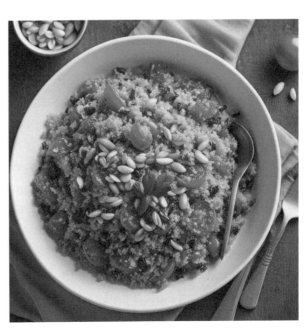

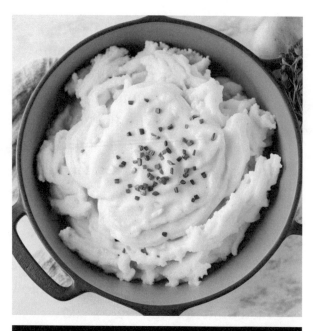

LOW-CALORIE MASHED POTATOES

PREP TIME: 5 minutes   COOK TIME: 15 minutes SERVES 6

Ingredients

- 2 pounds Yukon Gold potatoes, chopped into 1-inch cubes
- 1½ cups low-sodium chicken broth
- ¼ cup plain nonfat Greek yogurt
- 2 tablespoons chopped chives
- Salt
- Freshly ground black pepper

Directions

- Add the chicken stock and chopped potatoes to a medium pot set over high heat. Cover and bring to a boil. Reduce the heat to medium-high, cover, and simmer for ten minutes after the liquid begins to boil.
- Take the pot off of the hob. Don't drain the liquid. Season with salt and pepper, then add the yoghurt and chives. Mash the potatoes with a fork or potato masher until the texture you want is achieved.
- Remaining potatoes can be kept in the fridge for three to five days in an airtight container.

PER SERVING: Calories: 135; Total fat: 1g; Saturated fat: 0g; Sodium: 55mg; Carbohydrates: 28g; Fiber: 2g; Protein: 5g; Calcium: 33mg; Potassium: 698mg

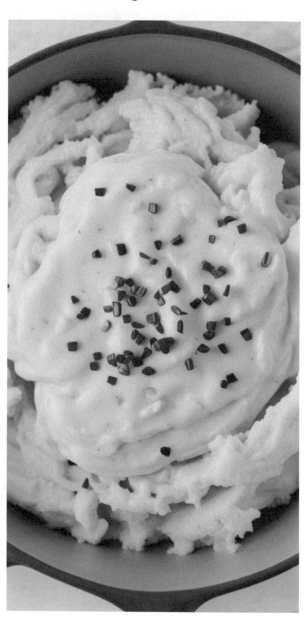

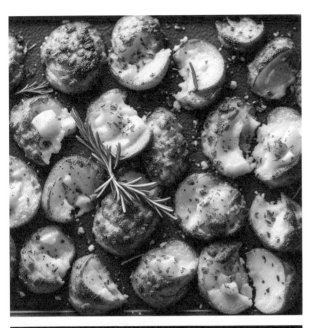

ROSEMARY-PARMESAN SMASHED POTATOES

PREP TIME: 5 minutes   **COOK TIME:** 30 minutes **SERVES 4**

Ingredients

- 1 pound baby potatoes
- 2 tablespoons olive oil
- 1 teaspoon crushed dried rosemary
- 1 teaspoon salt
- 1 teaspoon freshly ground black pepper
- 1 tablespoon Parmesan cheese

Directions

- Oven temperature: 450°F. Use nonstick aluminium foil or parchment paper to line a sheet pan.
- Put the potatoes in a microwave-safe bowl, pierce them twice or three times with a fork, and heat on high for five minutes until they are tender.
- On the sheet pan, arrange the potatoes two to three inches apart. Flatten the potatoes by gently pressing them down with a potato masher or the bottom of a mug. Sprinkle them with Parmesan cheese, salt, pepper, and rosemary after drizzling them with olive oil. Roast until crispy, 20 to 25 minutes.
- You may keep leftover potatoes in the fridge for up to four days.

PER SERVING: Calories: 152; Total fat: 7g; Saturated fat: 1g; Sodium: 611mg; Carbohydrates: 20g; Fiber: 3g; Protein: 3g; Calcium: 25mg; Potassium: 481mg

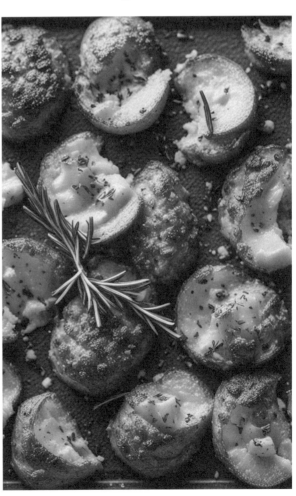

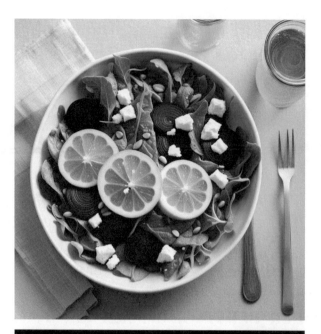

LEMON-SHALLOT CHAMPAGNE VINAIGRETTE

PREP TIME: 10 minutes MAKES 1 CUP

Ingredients

- ¼ cup champagne vinegar
- 1 tablespoon minced shallot
- 1 garlic clove, minced
- 1 teaspoon Dijon mustard
- Zest and juice of ½ lemon
- 1 tablespoon fresh thyme, or 1 teaspoon dried thyme
- ¾ cup extra-virgin olive oil
- Salt
- Freshly ground black pepper

Directions

- Whisk the vinegar, shallot, garlic, Dijon, lemon zest, lemon juice, and thyme in a small bowl.
- Season with salt and pepper after adding the oil. Mix the ingredients

- by whisking them together.
- For up to two weeks, keep the dressing refrigerated.

PER SERVING (2 TABLESPOONS):
Calories: 183; Total fat: 20g; Saturated fat: 3g; Sodium: 47mg; Carbohydrates: 1g; Fiber: 0g; Protein: 0g;
Calcium: 4mg; Potassium: 17mg

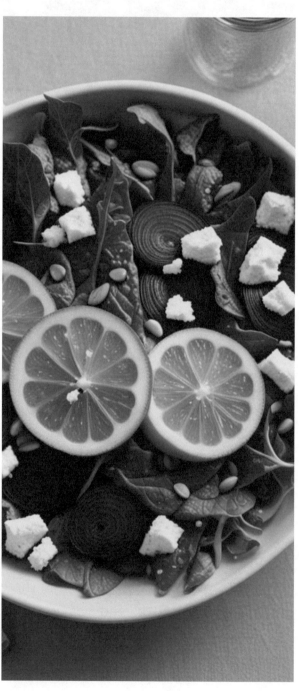

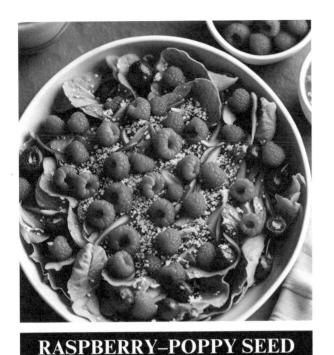

RASPBERRY–POPPY SEED DRESSING

PREP TIME: 5 minutes MAKES 1½ CUPS

Ingredients

- 1 cup fresh or defrosted frozen raspberries
- 6 tablespoons red wine vinegar
- 2 tablespoons honey
- 1 teaspoon ground mustard powder
- ½ cup avocado oil
- 1 teaspoon poppy seeds

Directions

- Put the raspberries, vinegar, honey, and mustard powder in a blender or food processor. Blend by pulsing until a liquid forms.
- As the mixture is processing, slowly pour in the avocado oil to mix it in.
- Transfer the dressing to an airtight jar. Shake to incorporate the poppy seeds.
- For up to two weeks, keep the dressing refrigerated.

PER SERVING (2 TABLESPOONS):
Calories: 100; Total fat: 9g; Saturated fat: 1g; Sodium: 1mg; Carbohydrates: 4g; Fiber: 1g; Protein: 0g; Calcium: 7mg; Potassium: 23mg

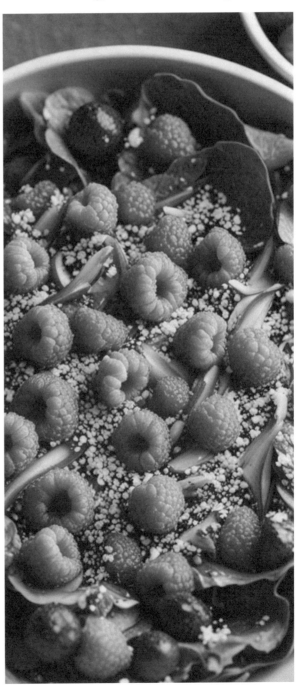

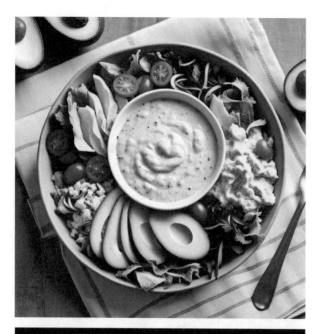

AVOCADO BUTTERMILK RANCH DRESSING

PREP TIME: 5 minutes MAKES 1½ CUPS

Ingredients

- 1¼ cups low-fat buttermilk
- 1 medium ripe avocado, peeled, pitted, and halved
- 1 garlic clove
- Juice of 1 lime
- 2 teaspoons onion powder
- 1 teaspoon dried chives
- 1 teaspoon dried parsley
- 1 teaspoon dried dill
- ½ teaspoon salt
- ½ teaspoon freshly ground black pepper

Directions

- Put the buttermilk, avocado, garlic, lime juice, onion powder, chives, parsley, dill, salt, and pepper in a blender or food processor. Blend by

- pulsing until a smooth liquid forms. Until you're ready to use it, chill.
- For up to a week, keep the dressing refrigerated in an airtight container.

PER SERVING (2 TABLESPOONS):
Calories: 40; Total fat: 3g; Saturated fat: 0g; Sodium: 147mg; Carbohydrates: 3g; Fiber: 1g; Protein: 1g; Calcium: 37mg; Potassium: 132mg

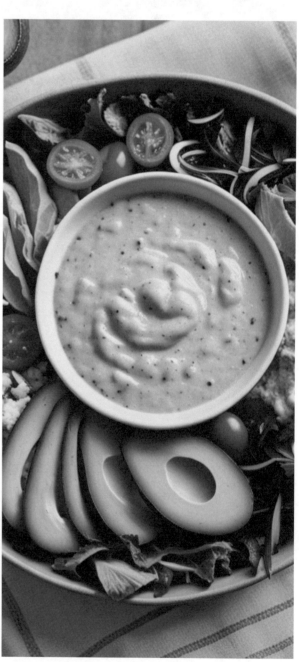

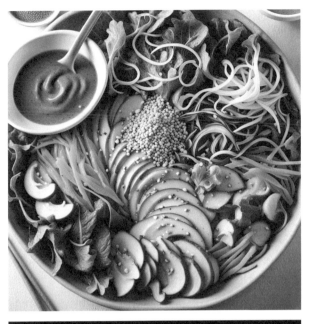

SESAME, MISO, AND GINGER DRESSING

PREP TIME: 5 minutes MAKES 1 CUP

Ingredients

- 2 tablespoons sesame oil
- ¼ cup avocado oil
- 3 tablespoons rice wine vinegar
- 2 tablespoons low-sodium soy sauce
- 1 garlic clove, quartered
- 1 (1-inch) piece fresh ginger, peeled and quartered (see Technique Trick)
- 1 tablespoon mirin or honey
- 1 tablespoon white miso
- 1 tablespoon sesame seeds

Directions

- Puree the sesame oil, avocado oil, vinegar, soy sauce, garlic, ginger, mirin, and miso in a food processor or blender until smooth. After moving the dressing to a container, add the sesame seeds and whisk.

- You can keep the dressing in the fridge for up to three or four weeks.

PER SERVING (2 TABLESPOONS):
Calories: 104; Total fat: 11g; Saturated fat: 1g; Sodium: 208mg; Carbohydrates: 1g; Fiber: 0g; Protein: 1g; Calcium: 4mg; Potassium: 24mg

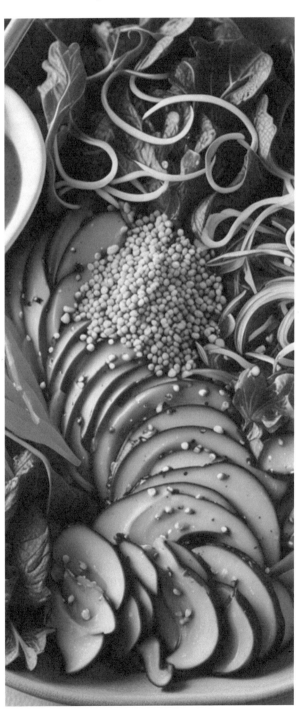

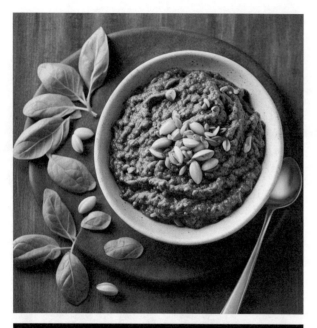

SPINACH-PISTACHIO PESTO SAUCE

PREP TIME: 10 minutes MAKES ½ CUP

Ingredients

- ½ cup baby spinach, firmly packed
- ½ cup fresh basil, firmly packed
- 1 garlic clove
- 2 tablespoons water, plus more as needed
- 3 tablespoons grated Parmesan cheese
- 2 tablespoons shelled pistachios, toasted
- 3 tablespoons extra-virgin olive oil

Directions

- Put the spinach, water, Parmesan cheese, pistachios, basil, and garlic in a food processor or blender. Pulse until a soft paste is formed.
- While blending, gradually add the oil and pulse until the consistency you want is achieved. Add another 1 to 2 tablespoons of water if you want a thinner sauce.
- The sauce can be frozen for up to six months or kept in the fridge for up to five days.

PER SERVING (1 TABLESPOON):
Calories: 65; Total fat: 6g; Saturated fat: 1g; Sodium: 36mg; Carbohydrates: 1g; Fiber: 0g; Protein: 1g;
Calcium: 23mg; Potassium: 40mg

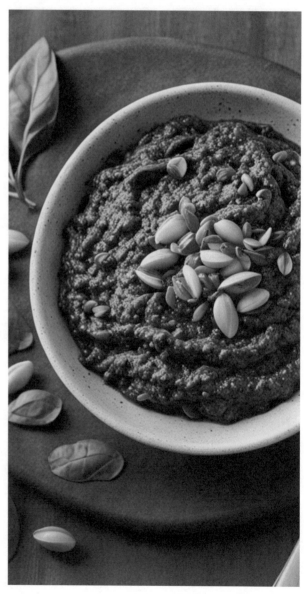

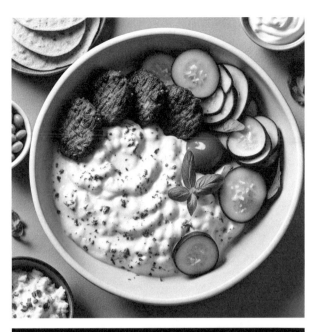

TZATZIKI SAUCE

PREP TIME: 5 minutes MAKES 1¼ CUPS

Ingredients

- ½ seedless English cucumber
- 1 cup plain nonfat Greek yogurt
- 1 tablespoon lemon juice
- 1 garlic clove
- ½ tablespoon extra-virgin olive oil
- 1 tablespoon fresh dill, or 1 teaspoon dried dill
- Salt
- Freshly ground black pepper

Directions

- Grate the cucumber with a box grater or in a food processor. After the cucumber has been grated, place it on a couple sheets of stacked paper towels, wrap it in them, and squeeze out any extra juice. Move the cucumber into a little bowl.
- Add the dill, oil, lemon juice, garlic, and Greek yoghurt to a food processor fitted with a chopping attachment. Add salt and pepper for seasoning. To blend, pulse.
- In the bowl containing the cucumber, add the dressing and whisk to mix. Until you're ready to use it, chill.
- Keep the sauce in the fridge for up to three days in an airtight container.

PER SERVING (2 TABLESPOONS): Calories: 24; Total fat: 1g; Saturated fat: 0g; Sodium: 24mg; Carbohydrates: 2g; Fiber: 0g; Protein: 3g; Calcium: 38mg; Potassium: 65mg

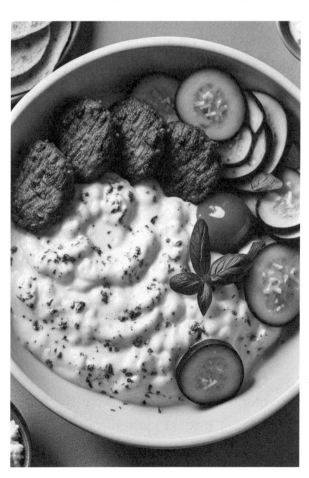

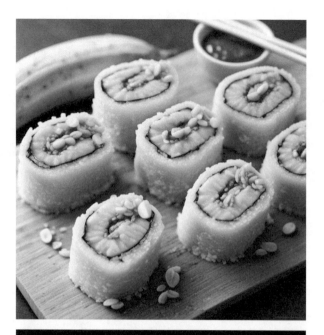

CRISPY BANANA SUSHI

PREP TIME: 5 minutes SERVES 1

Ingredients

- 1 (6-inch) whole-wheat tortilla
- 1 tablespoon almond butter
- 2 tablespoons puffed rice cereal
- 1 banana, peeled and whole
- Hemp seeds, for garnish (optional)

Directions

- Spread the almond butter on a flattened tortilla to coat it. Place a whole banana on one end of the tortilla after spreading the puffed rice cereal over the almond butter. Place the banana, almond butter, and puffed rice cereal inside the tortilla and roll it up tightly.
- Place the sushi slices with the banana facing up, then cut the rolled tortilla into ¾-inch slices. Top with hemp seeds and start eating right away.

PER SERVING: Calories: 377; Total fat: 16g; Saturated fat: 3g; Sodium: 213mg; Carbohydrates: 56g; Fiber: 12g; Protein: 11g; Calcium: 170mg; Potassium: 869mg

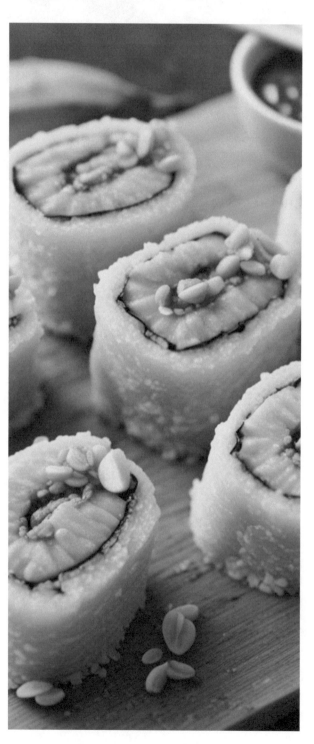

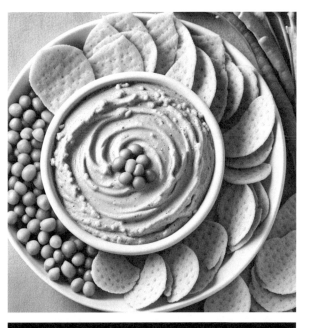

PEA HUMMUS

PREP TIME: 5 minutes MAKES 1 CUP

Ingredients

- 1 cup frozen peas, thawed
- 2 tablespoons tahini
- 3 garlic cloves
- 2 tablespoons lemon juice
- 1 teaspoon red pepper flakes, plus more for garnish (optional)
- ¼ teaspoon kosher salt, plus more for garnish
- ¼ teaspoon freshly ground black pepper, plus more for garnish
- 2 tablespoons extra-virgin olive oil, plus more for garnish

Directions

- Put the peas, tahini, lemon juice, garlic, red pepper flakes (if using), salt, and pepper in a blender or food processor. Pulse to mix, scraping down sides occasionally.
- Add the olive oil one tablespoon at a time while the processor is operating. Process until the consistency you want is achieved.
- Drizzle with extra olive oil, salt, pepper, and red pepper flakes (if using) just before serving.
- You may keep any leftover hummus in the fridge for up to a week.

PER SERVING (2 TABLESPOONS):
Calories: 69; Total fat: 5g; Saturated fat: 1g; Sodium: 78mg; Carbohydrates: 4g; Fiber: 1g; Protein: 2g; Calcium: 23mg; Potassium: 68mg

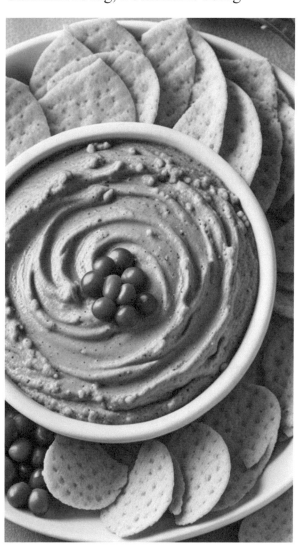

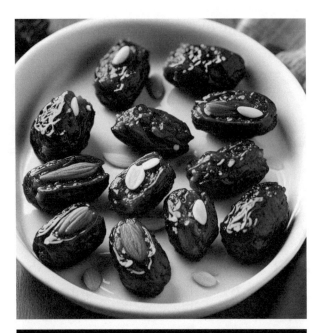

ALMOND-STUFFED DATES

PREP TIME: 5 minutes SERVES 4

Ingredients

- 8 Medjool dates, dried and pitted
- 4 tablespoons almond butter
- 8 whole raw almonds
- Sea salt, for garnish
- Mini chocolate chips, for garnish
- Ground cinnamon, for garnish

Directions

- Midway into the dates, make a lengthwise incision. Inside each date, spread ½ spoonful of almond butter. On top of the almond butter in the centre, place an almond. Add chocolate chips, ground cinnamon, and sea salt as garnish.
- Keep leftovers for up to a week at room temperature in an airtight container.

PER SERVING: Calories: 245; Total fat: 10g; Saturated fat: 1g; Sodium: 40mg; Carbohydrates: 40g; Fiber: 5g; Protein: 5g; Calcium: 93mg; Potassium: 471mg

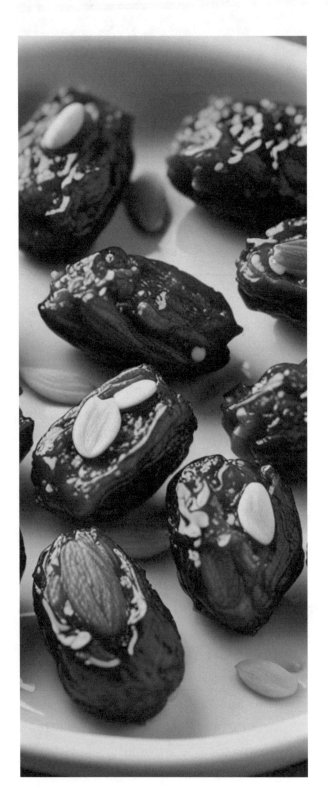

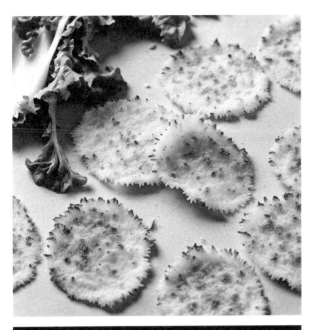

PARMESAN CRISPS

PREP TIME: 10 minutes   COOK TIME: 5 minutes SERVES 4

Ingredients

- Nonstick cooking spray
- 1 (4-ounce) block Parmesan cheese
- Freshly ground black pepper (optional)

Directions

- Oven temperature: 400°F. Spray cooking spray on a sheet pan after lining it with parchment paper.
- Using a zester or a box grater with tiny holes, finely shred the Parmesan cheese in a small bowl.
- On the parchment paper, use a tablespoon to form mounds of the Parmesan cheese. Then, using the back of the spoon, flatten the mounds, making sure they are at least 2 inches apart. Add pepper, if

used, as a garnish. Bake until golden, 5 to 8 minutes.
- Before removing off the parchment paper, let it cool. Savour it right now.
- Remaining food can be kept for up to three days at room temperature in an airtight container.

PER SERVING: Calories: 119; Total fat: 8g; Saturated fat: 4g; Sodium: 511mg; Carbohydrates: 4g; Fiber: 0g; Protein: 8g; Calcium: 242mg; Potassium: 51mg

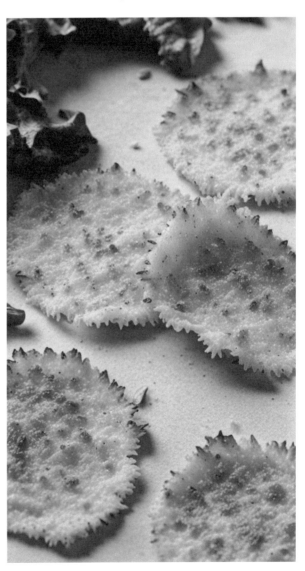

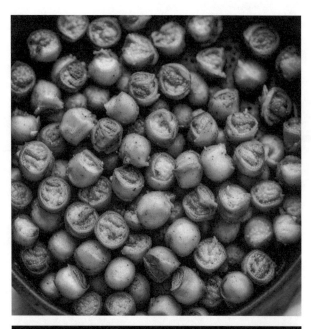

AIR FRYER–ROASTED RANCH CHICKPEAS

PREP TIME: 5 minutes   **COOK TIME: 20 minutes SERVES 2**

Ingredients

- 1 (15.5-ounce) can chickpeas, drained and rinsed
- 2 tablespoons dry buttermilk powder (see Cooking Hack)
- 2 teaspoons dried parsley
- 2 teaspoons onion powder
- 1 teaspoon dried chives
- ½ teaspoon garlic powder
- ¼ teaspoon dried dill
- ¼ teaspoon salt
- ¼ teaspoon freshly ground black pepper
- Nonstick cooking spray

Directions

- Spread the chickpeas out on a sheet pan covered with layers of paper towels to dry them. After patting dry with a second layer of paper towels, let it air dry for five minutes.
- Combine the buttermilk powder, parsley, onion powder, chives, garlic powder, dill, salt, and pepper in a small bowl to create the ranch spice blend. Put aside.
- Apply cooking spray to the air fryer basket. After spreading the dry chickpeas in the basket, fry them for five minutes at 400 degrees Fahrenheit.
- Add the chickpeas, cook for another 15 minutes, stirring every 5 minutes, until they are crisp and browned, and then spray them with cooking spray.
- Enjoy the cooked chickpeas right away after tossing them with 1 to 2 tablespoons of ranch seasoning blend.
- Keep any leftover chickpeas for up to a week at room temperature in an airtight container. To use with a subsequent batch of chickpeas, store any remaining ranch seasoning in an airtight container.

PER SERVING: Calories: 201; Total fat: 4g; Saturated fat: 1g; Sodium: 569mg; Carbohydrates: 32g; Fiber: 8g; Protein: 11g; Calcium: 142mg; Potassium: 272mg

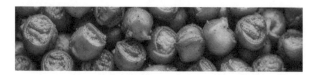

Week 1 Shopping List

Produce:
- 1 zucchini
- 3 bananas
- 1 mango
- 1 cauliflower
- 1 bag spinach
- 1 pint mixed berries
- 1 pint grape tomatoes
- 1 bag kale
- 1 head of romaine lettuce
- 1 cucumber
- Fresh mint
- Fresh basil
- Fresh parsley
- Fresh cilantro
- 1 lemon
- 1 lime
- 1 apple

Dairy & Alternatives:
- Nonfat milk (or preferred nondairy alternative)
- Plain nonfat Greek yogurt
- Kefir
- Cheddar cheese
- Mozzarella cheese
- Eggs

Grains & Seeds:
- Rolled oats
- Chia seeds
- Quinoa
- Whole-grain English muffins
- Almonds
- Walnuts
- Pecans

Nuts, Spices & Condiments:
- Cacao powder
- Cacao nibs
- Olive oil
- Maple syrup
- Ground flaxseed
- Honey
- Ground turmeric
- Ground cinnamon
- Ground ginger
- Red pepper flakes
- Kosher salt
- Black pepper

Pantry Essentials:
- Canned chickpeas
- Chicken or vegetable broth
- Whole-wheat tortillas (for wraps)

Days	Breakfast	Lunch	Snack	Dinner
Day 1	Chocolate-Zucchini Smoothie	Kale Caesar Salad	Almond-Stuffed Dates	Sheet Pan Veggie Hash
Day 2	Golden Milk Smoothie	Tangy No-Mayo Tuna Salad	Parmesan Crisps	Cauliflower Rice Burrito Bowl
Day 3	Acai Smoothie Bowl	Waldorf Chicken Salad Lettuce Wraps	Air Fryer-Roasted Ranch Chickpeas	Pesto Grain Bowl with Chickpeas
Day 4	Baked Oatmeal Cups	Beet, Goat Cheese, and Pistachio Salad	Pea Hummus with sliced veggies	Crispy Tofu Bowl
Day 5	Savory Pesto Oats	Watermelon, Tomato, Cucumber, Feta, and Mint Salad	Almond Butter & Banana Sweet Potato Toast	Salmon Teriyaki Power Bowl
Day 6	Spinach and Cheddar Almost Eggs Benedict	Grilled Halloumi Salad	Sunflower Taco Salad Bowl	Mushroom, Kale, and Feta Breakfast Tacos
Day 7	Baked Vegetable Frittata	Cold Sesame Noodle Bowl	Air Fryer–Roasted Ranch Chickpeas	Falafel Bowl

Week 2 Shopping List

Produce:
- 2 sweet potatoes
- 4 bananas
- 1 large avocado
- Mixed greens (for salads)
- 1 bag baby spinach
- 1 red bell pepper
- 1 cucumber
- 1 pint cherry tomatoes
- 1 bag arugula
- 1 head Bibb lettuce
- Fresh parsley
- Fresh cilantro
- Fresh thyme
- 1 lemon
- 1 lime

Dairy & Alternatives:
- Greek yogurt
- Cottage cheese
- Cheddar cheese
- Feta cheese
- Eggs

Grains & Seeds:
- Rolled oats
- Buckwheat flour
- Chia seeds
- Whole-wheat tortillas
- Quinoa
- Almonds

- Walnuts
- Sunflower seeds

Nuts, Spices & Condiments:
- Tahini
- Almond butter
- Honey
- Olive oil
- Dijon mustard
- Garlic powder
- Onion powder
- Salt & pepper
- Ground turmeric
- Ground cinnamon
- Chili powder
- Cumin

Pantry Essentials:
- Canned black beans
- Canned chickpeas
- Canned fire-roasted tomatoes with green chilies
- Brown rice
- Puffed rice cereal (for snacks)
- Whole-wheat panko breadcrumbs

Days	Breakfast	Lunch	Snack	Dinner
Day 1	Sweet Potato Toast with Almond Butter and Banana	Kale and Apple Salad with Walnuts	Crispy Banana Sushi	Cauliflower Risotto
Day 2	Buckwheat Pancakes with Berry Compote	Tangy No-Mayo Tuna Salad in Lettuce Wraps	Air Fryer-Roasted Ranch Chickpeas	Grilled Halloumi Salad with Arugula and Pomegranate
Day 3	Acai Smoothie Bowl	Kale Caesar Salad with Soft-Boiled Eggs	Parmesan Crisps	Cold Sesame Noodle Bowl with Edamame
Day 4	Savory Pesto Oats	Spinach and Cheddar Almost Eggs Benedict on Whole-Grain English Muffins	Pea Hummus with Cucumber Slices	Quinoa Salad with Cherry Tomatoes and Avocado
Day 5	Baked Oatmeal Cups with Cranberries and Pecans	Roasted Beet, Goat Cheese, and Pistachio Salad	Almond-Stuffed Dates with Sea Salt	Pesto Grain Bowl with Zucchini, Chickpeas, and Mozzarella
Day 6	Mushroom, Kale, and Feta Breakfast Tacos	Watermelon, Tomato, Cucumber, and Feta Salad	Air Fryer–Roasted Ranch Chickpeas	Falafel Bowl with Tzatziki Sauce
Day 7	Golden Milk Smoothie	Cauliflower Rice Burrito Bowl with Black Beans and Corn	Sunflower Taco Salad Bowl	Crispy Tofu Bowl with Jasmine Rice and Vegetables

Week 3 Shopping List

Produce:
- 3 bananas
- 2 avocados
- 1 large sweet potato
- 1 cucumber
- 1 pint cherry tomatoes
- 1 bag baby spinach
- 1 red bell pepper
- 1 bag mixed greens
- 1 bag shredded carrots
- Fresh basil
- Fresh parsley
- Fresh mint
- 1 lemon
- 1 lime

Dairy & Alternatives:
- Nonfat milk or preferred nondairy milk
- Greek yogurt
- Feta cheese
- Cottage cheese
- Eggs
- Cheddar cheese

Grains & Seeds:
- Rolled oats
- Whole-wheat tortillas
- Chia seeds
- Almonds
- Walnuts
- Sunflower seeds
- Quinoa
- Jasmine rice

Nuts, Spices & Condiments:
- Almond butter
- Olive oil
- Dijon mustard
- Honey
- Red pepper flakes
- Black pepper
- Kosher salt
- Cumin
- Ground turmeric
- Ground cinnamon
- Sesame seeds

Pantry Essentials:
- Canned black beans
- Canned chickpeas
- Whole-wheat panko breadcrumbs
- Vegetable broth
- Puffed rice cereal (for snacks)

Days	Breakfast	Lunch	Snack	Dinner
Day 1	Golden Milk Smoothie	Spinach and Feta Stuffed Wrap	Almond Butter & Banana on Sweet Potato Toast	Grilled Vegetable Quinoa Salad
Day 2	Chocolate-Zucchini Smoothie	Avocado and Black Bean Salad	Air Fryer–Roasted Ranch Chickpeas	Pesto Zoodles with Cherry Tomatoes and Parmesan
Day 3	Acai Smoothie Bowl	Kale Caesar Salad with Soft-Boiled Eggs	Almond-Stuffed Dates with Sea Salt	Falafel Bowl with Tzatziki and Fresh Herbs
Day 4	Sweet Potato Toast with Almond Butter and Banana	Tangy No-Mayo Tuna Salad	Crispy Banana Sushi	Mushroom, Kale, and Feta Tacos
Day 5	Buckwheat Pancakes with Berry Compote	Waldorf Chicken Salad in Lettuce Cups	Pea Hummus with Carrot Sticks	Cold Sesame Noodle Bowl with Edamame and Vegetables
Day 6	Savory Pesto Oats	Watermelon, Tomato, and Feta Salad	Parmesan Crisps	Cauliflower Rice Burrito Bowl with Black Beans and Corn
Day 7	Baked Oatmeal Cups with Cranberries and Pecans	Roasted Beet and Goat Cheese Salad with Arugula	Almond-Stuffed Dates with Cinnamon	Salmon Teriyaki Power Bowl with Brown Rice and Vegetables

Week 4 Shopping List

Produce:
- 3 bananas
- 1 large avocado
- 1 sweet potato
- 1 zucchini
- 1 bag mixed greens
- 1 cucumber
- 1 pint cherry tomatoes
- 1 bag baby spinach
- Fresh basil
- Fresh parsley
- Fresh cilantro
- Fresh thyme
- 1 lemon
- 1 lime

Dairy & Alternatives:
- Nonfat milk or preferred nondairy milk
- Greek yogurt
- Cottage cheese
- Cheddar cheese
- Feta cheese
- Eggs

Grains & Seeds:
- Rolled oats
- Whole-wheat tortillas
- Chia seeds
- Quinoa
- Jasmine rice

- Almonds
- Walnuts

Nuts, Spices & Condiments:
- Almond butter
- Olive oil
- Honey
- Ground turmeric
- Ground cinnamon
- Cumin
- Black pepper
- Kosher salt
- Red pepper flakes

Pantry Essentials:
- Canned black beans
- Canned chickpeas
- Vegetable broth
- Puffed rice cereal

Days	Breakfast	Lunch	Snack	Dinner
Day 1	Chocolate-Zucchini Smoothie	Avocado and Black Bean Salad	Pea Hummus with Carrot Sticks	Crispy Tofu Bowl with Jasmine Rice and Shredded Carrots
Day 2	Golden Milk Smoothie	Watermelon, Tomato, and Feta Salad	Almond-Stuffed Dates with Cinnamon	Cold Sesame Noodle Bowl with Edamame and Cucumbers
Day 3	Savory Pesto Oats	Spinach and Feta Stuffed Wrap	Air Fryer–Roasted Ranch Chickpeas	Grilled Vegetable Quinoa Salad with Basil
Day 4	Sweet Potato Toast with Almond Butter and Banana	Waldorf Chicken Salad Lettuce Wraps	Parmesan Crisps	Salmon Teriyaki Power Bowl with Brown Rice and Mixed Vegetables
Day 5	Buckwheat Pancakes with Berry Compote	Kale Caesar Salad with Soft-Boiled Eggs	Crispy Banana Sushi	Pesto Zoodles with Cherry Tomatoes and Parmesan
Day 6	Acai Smoothie Bowl	Tangy No-Mayo Tuna Salad	Pea Hummus with Sliced Bell Peppers	Cauliflower Rice Burrito Bowl with Black Beans and Corn
Day 7	Breakfast: Baked Oatmeal Cups with Cranberries and Pecans	Roasted Beet and Goat Cheese Salad with Arugula	Almond Butter & Banana on Sweet Potato Toast	Mushroom, Kale, and Feta Breakfast Tacos

Thank You

Thank you for choosing The Complete Obesity Fix Cookbook inspired by Dr. James DiNicolantonio's teachings. Your commitment to enhancing your health and well-being is commendable, and I am honoured that this book will be a part of your journey.

Creating this cookbook has been a labour of love, filled with passion for nutritious eating and the desire to empower individuals like you to make informed dietary choices. The recipes within these pages are designed not just to nourish your body but also to inspire a healthier lifestyle.

I hope you find joy in preparing these meals and discover new favourites that contribute to your journey toward better health. Your willingness to embrace change is truly inspiring, and I am excited for you to experience the benefits of these wholesome recipes.

Thank you for being part of this community dedicated to wellness. Here's to your health and happiness!

With appreciation,
Michelle C. Huff.

Made in United States
Cleveland, OH
15 January 2025

13442472R10042